Alive, Surviving Modern Oncology

Ann Gimpel

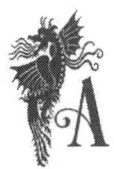

Contents

Acknowledgments	ix
Book Description	xiii
About the Cover	1
Author's Note	3
Introduction	9
1. Robert Nagourney, M.D. Interview	17
2. What Causes Cancer Anyway?	41
3. Karen's Story	55
4. Greg's Story	63
5. Ann's Story, Part 1	77
6. Peta's Story	83
7. Debbie's Story	89
8. Cancer is Big Business	93
9. Ann's Story, Part 2	107
10. Maria Wessling Bachteal's Story	117
11. Ann's Story, Part 3	123
12. Angela's Story	131
13. Vanessa's Story	143
14. Ann's Story, Part 4	153
15. Eleanor Hall's Story	161
16. Sharon Ann Merritt's Story	165
17. Ann's Story, Part 5	175
18. Lena Winslow's Story	183
19. The Good, The Bad, The Ugly	193
20. Noel Watson's Story	201
21. Mark Sean Taylor Interview	221
22. Amanda's Story	235

23. Ann's Story, Part 6	247
24. Dan Lyster's Story	255
25. Spiritual Pursuits	259
26. Nutrition	265
27. Integrative Oncology	279
Cancer Through Another Lens by Mark Lintern	287
Resources	309
Notes	319
About the Author	321
Also by Ann Gimpel	323

Copyright Page

All rights reserved.
Copyright © July 2023, Ann Gimpel
Cover by Ann Gimpel
Edited by Diane Eagle Kataoka
Names, characters, and incidents depicted in this book are products of the author's imagination or are used fictitiously. Any resemblance to actual events, locales, organizations, or people living or dead, is entirely coincidental and beyond the intent of the author.
No part of this book may be reproduced or shared by any electronic or mechanical means, including but not limited to printing, file sharing, e-mail, or web posting without written permission from the author.

Alive is dedicated to the Gerber Clinic in Reno, Nevada, and Sean Devlin, D.O., the integrative oncologist who gifted me with hope. It is also dedicated to every integrative care practitioner who puts patient care first and doesn't exist to fleece them out of their life savings.

I am grateful for the care I received from Dr. Devlin and the Gerber Clinic. They treated me with compassion. Dr. Devlin accepted me as a full partner in my treatment rather than pushing anything down my throat. He had opinions but also valued mine.

When I told him I was going to write Alive, he laughed and said, "Heaven help us all."

Acknowledgments

I'd like to extend a personal note of thanks to everyone who contributed to Alive. Far beyond the survivors who were willing to share their stories, others in the integrative cancer community were forthcoming with their support and knowledge.

Special thanks to Abbey Mitchell, the founder and administrator of Healing Cancer Study and Support group for allowing me to troll for stories on her Facebook group. Her enthusiasm for this project has been heartwarming.

In a vast departure from infusion centers and traditional oncology clinics that tend to be chilly and sterile, the online integrative care cancer community has been warm and welcoming. I've learned so much since I began writing this book and have gathered skills and strategies. It's far more empowering than, "Let's just wait to see if the chemo works..."

"Just waiting" places one in a passive role, not the best place to be. Dealing with cancer, or any serious illness, has a strong mental component. We must be active partners in every aspect of our care. The online community became my partners. I found people who cared about me, who had ongoing suggestions to make my journey richer.

Maria Wessling Bachteal went above and beyond. The resource section is as thorough as it is because of her far-ranging wisdom and many years of experience in nutrition and the integrative/alternative care cancer field.

One of my contributors, Greg Smith from Hong Kong, has been exceedingly helpful sending me research articles, which have spawned ideas.

Alive is not an original scientific work. Rather it's a compilation of ideas and research gleaned from untold hours of Internet searches. Special thanks to Sam Apple, who generously allowed me to excerpt from his article, *An Old Idea Revived: Starve Cancer to Death* that appeared in the 5/12/2016 issue of the New York Times Magazine.

Thanks as well to John Horgan who kindly agreed to let me use large portions of his article, *The Cancer Industry: Hype Versus Reality*, that appeared in the 2/12/2020 issue of Scientific American.

Mark Lintern was a hard fellow to track down, but once I did, he gave me permission to reproduce, *Cancer Through Another Lens*, the product of eight years of his research.

Bits and pieces from many research articles are also quoted with full citations so you can look up things that interest you.

Special thanks to my longtime friend, hiking buddy, and ace editor, Diane Eagle Kataoka. She volunteered her time editing this project because she believed in its importance.

I'd be remiss to not mention my husband. I can knock out a novel in six weeks. *Alive* took months. I agonized over it in ways I never do over fiction. His steadfast support has been both welcome and amazing. He's been by my side throughout my cancer saga. I couldn't have done any of this without him.

Apologies if I left anyone out. It wasn't intentional.

What began as a lonely endeavor turned into so much more.

Book Description

Cancer is a bitch of a disease. Every single person who's experienced being diagnosed and treated is a hero. There are a lot of cancer books out there. What's different about this one?

Maybe nothing. Maybe a lot. I'm a psychologist by trade. About fifteen years back, I started writing novels. Unfortunately, there's not a scrap of fiction in *Alive*. There are also no dragons, unicorns, or magical worlds. This book was tough to write. In places, it will be equally tough to read. In addition to my personal saga, it includes stories from other brave souls who volunteered to be part of this project. There are also chapters about the etiology of cancer, cancer as big business in America (and elsewhere), avoiding scams, and integrative oncology.

Like most, I started my cancer journey believing the MDs had my best interests at heart. A few did, but to so many others I was nothing but a number, a statistic, many steps removed from a human being.

My hope for *Alive* is it will empower others to stand up for themselves, to ask questions, to do their own research. Ultimately, everyone's life is precious and worth the effort of self-advocacy.

About the Cover

I don't normally make my own covers, but I knew precisely what I wanted for this one. The red and blue are an artistic rendition of arteries and veins. Some contributors to *Alive* viewed the red as a baptism by fire. The caduceus symbolizes the Hippocratic Oath that all newly minted doctors take when they, among other things, vow to "do no harm."

Author's Note

This book is intensely personal for me. It details my cancer journey as I've wended my way through the challenges of the American oncology treatment system. Writing it was cathartic since so many unfortunate events ensued over the years since my diagnosis.

Along the way, I discovered many oncologists aren't interested in patients with opinions, patients who ask questions, or patients who research things on their own. God forbid you take supplements or try to block any of cancer's many metabolic pathways. I've lived through a botched surgery, a second surgery to fix problems created by the first, surgeons who lied to me, an infusion center that fired me, a specialist who ghosted me.

The list is long.

I've also met some stellar human beings who treated me with courtesy, dignity, and respect. The bar was low, I'm telling you, damned low. I was pathetically grateful for every scrap of attention that reinforced my humanity. We are more than statistics and expiration dates. Perhaps a decade (or two) of oncology practice drums that out of some doctors.

As I sit at the front end of this writing project, I have no idea how long it will take or how many pages the finished product will be. Long enough to tell my story. Other people's stories too. As they say, it takes a village. If *Alive* only chronicled my story, you could chalk it up to me having bad luck.

A whole lot of bad luck, but bad luck, nonetheless.

An idealistic part of me wishes it were true. But I'm far from the only cancer patient who's been treated abysmally by MDs and clinics. Subpar treatment appears to be far more prevalent than I ever expected. It makes me sad because it doesn't have to be like that.

When I refer to "standard of care" treatment, what I mean is treatment signed, sealed, and recognized by boarded oncologists. Integrative treatment can incorporate standard of care, but it goes much further and encompasses a whole person approach.

If *Alive* helps even one other person navigate answers for their own cancer diagnosis, it will have been worth the time it took me to write my portions and organize the rest of the book into a meaningful whole. Cancer patients only have one opportunity to get the right chemo or immunotherapy drug (or other indicated treatment). If they're given the wrong compound out of the gate because "we give everyone with your cancer X and Y," that incorrect treatment could wreak havoc with future response to much of anything.

Not that a patient can't survive if they get a chemo agent that is ineffective for first-line treatment, but that ineffective agent will have a negative effect on the body as a whole and make it tougher for future interventions to find success.

If you want a cure—and who doesn't?—you need to get it right the first time. "Right" requires genomic or molecular testing most oncologists aren't willing to offer unless you ask for it. Even if you do, chances are you'll get a lot of flak. Many patients have been told, "Insurance won't pay for it" (not true, it oftentimes will). Or, "Why would you want that? It won't change anything."

In the "we give everyone with your cancer X and Y world," no, it won't change a thing. But that's not the kind of treatment you want or deserve.

My observation is doctors will offer genomic/molecular testing—after a patient experiences a recurrence. This is akin to shutting the barn door once the horse is long gone.

Finding a practitioner who listens to you, includes you in all treatment decisions, and values your input is key. Doctors need to go to bat for you with insurance companies and be your advocate for treatments that might not be readily forthcoming.

Physicians who go that extra mile are worth gold.

My claim to fame is as a fictional author. I have well over a hundred novels to my credit. Within the coming pages, you won't find a single dragon or unicorn or shifter. No mythical worlds. No battle scenes. No slow-burn romance.

What you will find is up close and personal and raw. I've been ridden hard and put away wet. My tale is far from unique. So many professionals, the ones who took the Hippocratic Oath to "Do No Harm" aren't invested in exceptional patient care. This is harsh, but they appear to care about not getting sued. So, they practice cookie-cutter medicine whether it's indicated in a particular case or not. That way, whatever they did—or didn't do—will vindicate them in court regardless of patient outcomes.

I'm a psychologist by trade. I spent years working hand-in-glove with MDs in clinics. For a time, I taught behavioral medicine at a family practice residency. It gave me a decent snapshot of the medical profession, but nothing like I received as a cancer patient. For the most part, the family medicine doctors at the residency cared deeply about quality patient care. They went the extra mile and did adequate research. They asked a lot of questions.

And did their best to find answers to questions fielded by their patients.

By contrast, many of the oncologists I ran into seemed bored, disinterested, disconnected, indifferent. The one I thought actually cared about me ended up ghosting me. Another ushered me out of her office less than five minutes into my prepared list of questions. During a previous visit, she spent much of our session time talking about herself, her interests, her child who'd just started college...

The part she didn't get was I was there in her office to talk about my life. Mine. Why would I not do research and have questions? As the resident expert, she should have at least tried to answer them rather than making it clear I was a pain in her rump.

Or talking about herself.

Alrighty. Here we go. What happened to me, and the lessons I learned, will be interspersed with other people's cancer stories. Sometimes my story will be hard to read. Apologies up front for that. It was even harder to live. Maybe, through writing it all down, the ghosts residing in my head will finally be laid to rest.

My fond hope for this project is a bit self-serving. If I'm successful, I won't keep reliving the horrors that have peppered the last two-and-a-half years. Beyond that, if this book helps even one other cancer patient stand up for themselves, the effort will have been worth it.

Here's the caveat: Nothing in this book should be construed as medical advice. I am not an MD. What's contained in these pages are simply my opinions and the opinions of those who contributed stories, interviews, and other material to *Alive*. You will agree with some viewpoints and disagree with others. Still, I hope there's enough of value to keep you reading.

Cancer is a complex topic. I'd be worse than a fool to claim I had all the answers, or even most of them. Nope. I've barely scratched the surface.

No path open to cancer patients is without risk. Choosing standard of care treatment is far from a guarantee of success. On the other hand, neither is choosing integrative care. In an ideal world, you could blend the two approaches, but most standard of care oncologists want nothing to do with integrative care.

As the saying goes, you spin the wheel and take your chances. A critical element is you have to believe in the path you've chosen. We all possess an innate wisdom about our bodies. Trust your instincts. They won't steer you wrong. Visualizing outcomes is a proven strategy. It truly does work.

Wishing you all love and light as you find your way.

Introduction

I grew up in the 1950s, a daughter of Russian immigrant stock. This particular wave of immigrants prioritized education over everything. I knew I was going to college before I hit kindergarten. It was that bad.

My parents wanted me to be a doctor. By their way of thinking, it was the highest star in the sky, and the one their daughter should shoot for. I tried. Honest I did. I took all the science classes that were precursors to being accepted into medical school, but medicine never sang to me.

I still remember the start of my junior year at University of Washington when I had to declare a major. Back then, nothing much was computerized. Computers took up entire floors of buildings, and you talked to them by feeding them punch cards.

There I was, with the catalog of potential majors open across my lap. As I paged through it, I kept returning to psychology, and eventually declared it as my major with a minor in English and another in history.

My parents were devastated.

How could I ever earn a living, they asked, wringing their hands.

I was twenty years old, and while feeding myself was high on my list, I realized how little I could get by on. I didn't need my father's income (he was a dentist). Neither did I plan to "marry well" so someone else could take care of me.

The 1960s were freeing in many ways. Women's traditional roles were replaced by a generation of females for whom the sky was the limit.

I was one of them.

I finished my B.S. in three years and moved out to the Olympic Peninsula to live in a commune with a bunch of good folks. We were convinced we were going to change the world. If someone had told us we'd eventually turn into clones of our parents, we'd have been horrified.

It's precisely what happened to so many of us.

Me included.

After my unauthorized (the parental perspective) year off, I became a good daughter once again and attended University of the Pacific. After an M.A. in psychology there, I enrolled in UC Davis. Their doctoral program in physiological psychology was (ahem) far closer to the medical career I'd eschewed than I was willing to admit, but I loved it.

Davis housed one of the nation's seven regional primate centers, so we had monkeys to experiment on along with cats, mice, rats, ground squirrels, and a few other unrelated species. One of my fellow grad students kept fish tanks.

I may not have been a med student, but as a teaching assistant, I taught many premeds. Several ended up sobbing in my office because the grade they assumed they'd receive in my class would kill their chances of moving forward. I told them to party less and study more. Got a bunch of dirty looks.

Med school has always been competitive to get into.

That part has never changed.

Roll the clock forward a few years. Okay, a whole lot of years. I ended up returning to school in the late 1980s and obtained a Ph.D. in clinical psychology along with a license to practice.

That career path landed me in a chronic pain rehab clinic for several years and teaching at a family medicine residency program for several more. I worked hand-in-glove with MDs during those years. Many of my closest friends are doctors.

I wanted to put that out there in case some of you wonder how I came to hate MDs as you read through *Alive*. I don't hate them. Nothing could be further from the truth. I feel sorry for many of them. Medicine hasn't been the golden ring they'd hoped for from the day they began their formal training.

As with anyone living a tarnished dream, some MDs have become withdrawn, bitter. Where compassion and openness would serve them, they've chosen to hide behind their white coats. I have no idea how oncologists deal with the cavalcade of deaths.

Certainly not by embracing any of the integrative options that might improve their patients' quality of life. Or, God forbid, integrative treatments that have a solid track record of keeping patients alive.

What do I mean by that? It's been documented since the 1920s that sugar feeds cancer (Warburg effect). If you wander into any infusion center, what do you see? Cookies, crackers, sandwiches on white bread, applesauce, candy, cookies, cake, soda, juice. Everything on the above list is loaded with sugar and shouldn't be part of any eating plan for cancer patients.

Simply altering the food that's offered at infusion centers would give patients a better shot at remaining alive. I remember having that discussion with the supervising nurse at the infusion center where I briefly received treatment. When I mentioned they might want to substitute Ka'Chava for Boost and Ensure, she looked it up and told me it was far too expensive.

There it is. What your life is worth to them.

They collect tens of thousands for chemo infusions but aren't willing to put themselves out to provide healthy snacks. Ka'Chava does cost more than Boost, but it's real food made with quality ingredients. Boost and Ensure are sugar mixed with chemicals, vitamins, and food coloring.

Back to oncologists and death. I produced a standard set of lectures when I taught at the residency. One of them was

"Giving Bad News." A large part of that lecture was dealing with your own emotions around patients whose death was imminent.

Pro hint: walling yourself off from your feelings isn't a preferred approach.

I went into my cancer journey trusting my care providers. That phase didn't last long. I have the utmost respect for anyone who has the guts to admit they don't know something. Even more for MDs who welcome you as partners in your own care.

Some doctors breeze through that gauntlet. They have no problem saying, "Gosh, I'm not sure, but I'll research it for you." Others would rather fall on their swords. So, I got a bunch of doublespeak. One doctor ushered me out of her office in the middle of my third question. I'd driven three hours to see her, waited 30 minutes in her waiting room, and she'd given me a whopping five minutes before dismissing me.

That's just rude.

We'll call her Dr. Kick-Em-When-They're-Down. She ended up firing me (big surprise). More on her later.

In so many ways, my cancer journey has been a wakeup call.

I'm sure there are decent oncologists out there but finding them isn't easy. How do I know? I belong to several online cancer groups, traditional and integrative, and my experiences are far from unique.

It's a good lead-in to the structure of this book.

My story will weave among stories from other survivors. Other than formatting, I've left their stories intact, in their voices. Many hurt my heart to read. When I floated the idea of including stories beyond my own, I thought perhaps a handful of survivors would want to participate.

The response has been overwhelming. Because I refused to turn anyone down, there are many stories. Some mix traditional treatment with integrative care. Others are integrative straight down the line. Many mirror my own journey where their starting point was traditional care, and then they branched out for various reasons.

I hope you read them with an open mind and heart. Take a few moments to digest each story after you've read it. Unless you've been there, no one truly understands on a visceral level what it's like to be told you have cancer. It changes everything in one split second. The survivors who contributed to *Alive* are brave souls.

Generous men and women who, like me, hope their experiences can help someone else. Some wanted me to share their names; others preferred their first names only.

In addition to survivor stories, I've included chapters on related topics including cancer as big business, current theories about the etiology of cancer, the importance of including some sort of spiritual practice, integrative oncology, nutrition, and interviews from kind and gracious people who have become leaders in the field of cancer care.

In the back of *Alive* I'm including an appendix of resources. Keep in mind, they're fluid. The further out from *Alive's* publication date we get, the more likely some of them will no longer be available.

My second caveat is this. There are a whole lot of integrative care clinics and practitioners out there. Unfortunately, many of them are not on the up and up. Nope. They milk funds out of dying, desperate people. A chapter later in this book titled "The Good, The Bad, The Ugly" talks about scams.

How can you tell the difference between a decent clinic and one that isn't?

It's not easy. If possible, talk with others who've received treatment at a clinic you're considering. This goes for traditional oncology as well. Finding satisfied patients is important. The next step is joining a few integrative/alternative care online groups. Find ones that don't espouse any particular approach. Healing Cancer Study and Support group on Facebook is excellent. It has close to 20,000 members and a deep files section where you can research various treatments to discover if there's actually science standing behind them.

I've never yet floated a question to that group where someone didn't have an answer.

Most research is conducted on the new million-dollar-baby wonder drugs. Big surprise since they're where Big Pharma cashes in. In a later chapter, we'll talk about how cancer is a huge and lucrative business in America and elsewhere. But there is research on many integrative care strategies and interventions, too. For example, the Riordan Clinic has a number of papers about intravenous Vitamin C. Dr. Isaac Eliaz has published many papers on modified citrus pectin. There are scads of podcasts, articles in PubMed, and in prestigious journals as well chronicling the efficacy of integrative care.

Beginning your research will feel daunting. Cancer isn't something any of us ever wanted to become an expert on, or even conversant with.

Your journey will take time, but your life is worth it.

Let's get started, shall we?

To set the tone for the rest of the book, I'm leading out with an interview I conducted with Robert Nagourney, M.D.

Robert Nagourney, M.D. Interview

Biographical Information:

Robert A. Nagourney, MD, is Medical and Laboratory Director of The Nagourney Cancer Institute in Long Beach, California, and an Associate Clinical Professor at University of California Irvine. He is board certified in internal medicine, medical oncology, and hematology.

A native of Bridgeport, Connecticut, Dr. Nagourney completed undergraduate education at Boston University, earning a BA in Chemistry, Summa Cum Laude, Phi Beta Kappa with Distinction in Biochemistry. He received his MD at McGill University in Montreal, Canada, where he was a University Scholar. After completing his residency in Internal Medicine at the University of California, Irvine, Dr. Nagourney received fellowship training in Medical Oncology at Georgetown University in Washington, DC, and went on to complete a second fellowship in hematology at the Scripps Institute in La Jolla,

California, where he was the recipient of the Scripps Institute Young Investigator Award.

After serving as the Medical Director of the Todd Cancer Institute, Dr. Nagourney later went on to found The Nagourney Cancer Institute, a cancer research center located in Long Beach, California, that has pioneered the development of "functional profiling" in human tumors. This platform uses human tumor biopsies in tissue culture to measure the effect of chemotherapy drugs and combinations to select treatments for cancer patients. This has proven highly effective for the prediction of clinical response to therapy before treatment is administered. Success with cytotoxic drugs has led to the study of "targeted" agents and more recently agents that effect cellular metabolism as cancer therapeutics. This was the topic of Dr. Nagourney's highly acclaimed TEDx talk.

With over 20 years' experience in human tumor primary culture analyses, Dr. Nagourney has authored more than 100 manuscripts, book chapters and abstracts including publications in the Journal of Clinical Oncology, Gynecological Oncology, and The Journal of National Cancer Institute. As co-investigator on national cooperative trials, Dr. Nagourney is recognized for the introduction of Platin/Gemcitabine doublets to the treatment of advanced ovarian and breast cancer. In 2015 he was the recipient of the NAACP "Trailblazer In Medicine" Award. As the author of the 2013 book "Outliving Cancer," Dr. Nagourney is a frequently invited lecturer for numerous professional organizations and universities. He has served as a reviewer and is on the editorial boards of several journals including Clinical Cancer Research, British Journal of Cancer, Gynecologic

Oncology, Cancer Research, and the *Journal of Medicinal Food*. Dr Nagourney resides in Long Beach, California with his wife.

Interview

Ann: You're traditionally trained and boarded as an oncologist and hematologist and also in internal medicine. What made you decide to branch out and take a different approach to cancer than your peers?

Dr. Nagourney: I started my undergraduate studies and received a degree in chemistry. I then went on to complete my medical degree and graduated from McGill University in Montreal. From there, I did not one but two fellowships. One was at Georgetown University in solid tumor oncology with a focus on pancreatic and gastrointestinal malignancies. Before that, I had completed a residency in California. It was a bit of culture shock to move from Montreal to California.

I returned to California to complete my second fellowship in hematology. So I had a broad exposure to cancer medicine, but I started quite early in my career working in a research laboratory. Even when I was a first and second year medical student, I was making rounds and hobnobbing with medical oncologists and fellows. I became quite friendly with the senior staff and faculty.

I got a birds eye view of cancer medicine going into the 70s and 80s, and it was pretty dismal. Although the response rates to interventions weren't great, the basic research opportunities were quite striking. And so I doubled back into oncology after not expecting to be there once I'd published some papers in the field.

I returned to oncology, finished my fellowship at Georgetown, and I was all the time, all the while, wondering why we were not making more headway in the field, particularly as a fellow. I actually wrote a book called *Outliving Cancer*. In the book, I described my experiences as a fellow.

I had come into my fellowship having been a very accomplished resident. I was the go-to guy for the arterial lines, the chest tubes, the intubation. I could figure out the complex cases. But when I got to my oncology fellowship, everybody died miserably. No matter how hard I tried, I couldn't seem to right the ship. And I wondered if we were doing this right.

I was certain we were missing something. So I moved to my second fellowship where hematologic cases were more responsive. I had recently met an investigator out of NIH who was convinced that if we studied cancer cell death in a laboratory model, we could predict outcomes. This was in the 1980s at a time when everyone hated the concept of human tissue studies.

For many years, people had tried to study human cancer in a test tube and predict outcomes. So I was stepping into a field where most people would have told me to stay away. But it worked. I couldn't deny the efficacy of the treatments we were identifying. I questioned why everyone hated this field when it worked, and I realized we'd been going about it all wrong.

Most people believe cancer is a disease of cell growth. As a result, cancer cells must be stopped from growing. That's what most of the drugs we use are designed to do. So I thought, well

Oncology, Cancer Research, and the *Journal of Medicinal Food*. Dr Nagourney resides in Long Beach, California with his wife.

Interview

Ann: You're traditionally trained and boarded as an oncologist and hematologist and also in internal medicine. What made you decide to branch out and take a different approach to cancer than your peers?

Dr. Nagourney: I started my undergraduate studies and received a degree in chemistry. I then went on to complete my medical degree and graduated from McGill University in Montreal. From there, I did not one but two fellowships. One was at Georgetown University in solid tumor oncology with a focus on pancreatic and gastrointestinal malignancies. Before that, I had completed a residency in California. It was a bit of culture shock to move from Montreal to California.

I returned to California to complete my second fellowship in hematology. So I had a broad exposure to cancer medicine, but I started quite early in my career working in a research laboratory. Even when I was a first and second year medical student, I was making rounds and hobnobbing with medical oncologists and fellows. I became quite friendly with the senior staff and faculty.

I got a birds eye view of cancer medicine going into the 70s and 80s, and it was pretty dismal. Although the response rates to interventions weren't great, the basic research opportunities were quite striking. And so I doubled back into oncology after not expecting to be there once I'd published some papers in the field.

I returned to oncology, finished my fellowship at Georgetown, and I was all the time, all the while, wondering why we were not making more headway in the field, particularly as a fellow. I actually wrote a book called *Outliving Cancer*. In the book, I described my experiences as a fellow.

I had come into my fellowship having been a very accomplished resident. I was the go-to guy for the arterial lines, the chest tubes, the intubation. I could figure out the complex cases. But when I got to my oncology fellowship, everybody died miserably. No matter how hard I tried, I couldn't seem to right the ship. And I wondered if we were doing this right.

I was certain we were missing something. So I moved to my second fellowship where hematologic cases were more responsive. I had recently met an investigator out of NIH who was convinced that if we studied cancer cell death in a laboratory model, we could predict outcomes. This was in the 1980s at a time when everyone hated the concept of human tissue studies.

For many years, people had tried to study human cancer in a test tube and predict outcomes. So I was stepping into a field where most people would have told me to stay away. But it worked. I couldn't deny the efficacy of the treatments we were identifying. I questioned why everyone hated this field when it worked, and I realized we'd been going about it all wrong.

Most people believe cancer is a disease of cell growth. As a result, cancer cells must be stopped from growing. That's what most of the drugs we use are designed to do. So I thought, well if cancer cell growth is the target, we've been testing drugs that stop growth.

It's the principle behind chemo-sensitivity. Can we introduce a drug and stop cells from proliferating? They used different endpoints: thymidine incorporation, DNA synthesis, clonogenicity, growth to confluence. There were all these growth, growth, growth endpoints. Not a one of them predicted outcomes. In fact, there was an editorial published in the early 80s in the New England Journal of Medicine that said the field was dead.

That was exactly when I was getting interested in it. I realized we were testing something very different. We were testing why cells die when they were supposed to, not stop growing but die. At the time, I didn't completely understand what I was doing, but I knew it worked. So I thought, well if we are measuring cell death and it's predictive, then is it possible cancer isn't really driven by growth? Is it possible cancer is a different animal?

I began to dig into that. I went to Amsterdam to give some papers and I came across a very interesting study in the early 90s about the phenomenon of apoptosis: programmed cell death. It changed my life overnight.

I realized suddenly that my measurements in my test tubes were, in fact, measuring something very important and fundamental about the biology of cancer and that everyone else had missed the exit. They had gone right past cell death to cell growth inhibition, and it had failed.

So I said, if we're measuring cell death, then this should predict outcomes. And we set about publishing a series of papers on leukemia that were highly successful. It's interesting because our published series date back to the 1980s, but no one wanted to read them. No one wanted to publish them. No one wanted to test them because they were all quite convinced that the field of human tumor primary culture wouldn't work.

We realized we had something that actually worked. The medical oncology community were completely unwilling to listen. I went to Toronto to give a paper on leukemia. That didn't engender any interest. We published papers on drug resistance reversal that didn't get any interest. I identified the first successful treatment for patients with hairy cell leukemia. That didn't get any interest. I published the first paper for triple negative breast cancer, and I published the first paper on treatment for refractory ovarian cancer. None of them received any interest.

It was obvious we were confronting a medical oncology community characterized by denialism. They were not going to be convinced no matter what we said. And I thought what I needed to do was go out and prove this. So, we did. We wrote protocols for the Gynecologic Oncology Group (GOG), a national cooperative group funded by the National Cancer Institute.

Philip DeSaia, was a friend, colleague, and chairman of the GOG. But even he had a difficult time promoting what I was doing, even though he clearly believed in it. The problem is we have an entrenched establishment that has no interest in changing what they do. Period. No matter how good your data, no matter how compelling your science, they're just not going to listen.

One of the stories was very interesting. We wrote, conducted, and prepared to publish a national clinical trial, showcasing a drug combination I had invented in my laboratory. The paper was successful. In fact, at the time we submitted the paper for publication, the results of our study provided the longest survivorship in platinum resistant ovarian cancer in the history of the GOG. They refused to publish the paper. We went from journal to journal to journal and kept getting turned down.

You have to understand, this was an NCI funded, GOG, phase 2 trial. We're not talking about some fly-by-night idea I came up with overnight. This was a national trial. They didn't want to publish it because the results were much better than their results. That meant what we did worked, and they were not going to hear about it.

So I had to go back to Phil DeSaia, my ally, and tell him his organization was refusing to publish an NCI funded cooperative group, GOG trial. He said, "Okay, I'll take care of this."

Next thing, Gynecologic Oncology published the study. So we were the first ever to prove that a treatment that's used today around the world worked. The fact that we found it using a human tumor primary culture 3D organoid system, was not something they wanted to hear about.

That is an example of the denialism that is a characteristic of the modern oncologic community. The fact that what we do works better is of no interest to them.

Low dose chemotherapy is a little bit of a slippery slope. We published our paper in GOG with a relatively low dose chemotherapy regimen. And we did pioneer using appropriate low doses, but you have to be careful. There are some who practice very low doses, and that can be hazardous because it basically telescopes your punch, and it allows the tumor to develop resistance that might otherwise not occur. What we're looking for in modern oncology isn't maximum tolerated dose but minimum effective dose. There is a difference. That's where we work. I have the luxury of picking substances that will work, so I can use reasonable doses rather than bludgeoning patients with chemotherapy.

For the most part, genomic platforms haven't predicted outcomes. Gene profiles are static measures of genetic elements. It's a little bit like trying to live in a blueprint. It's a general guideline of what you're going to build, but you don't get a feel for the building until you walk around in it. It's why people who develop properties for sale always build a model so you can walk around and see what the building feels like. That's human tumor primary culture analysis. It's a real hands-on feel for what's going on with the tumor, not simply a blueprint.

Ann: You founded your cancer institute 20 years ago. In that time, have you adjusted or refined your approach? If so, what changes have you made?

Dr. Nagourney: Initially, before the current institute was established, we studied human hematologic malignancies. My earliest papers were on chronic leukemia The reason we used those was because, in a pure tissue culture environment, we were looking for pure cellular material. At the time, I was convinced about the genomic revolution. So I wanted to do gene analysis, perform electrophoretic studies, and study gene phenomena. I wanted to look at cancer through the lens of modern genomics.

So I wanted a pure tissue culture. We were using CLL and used different techniques to obtain pure cultures. The trouble was most people don't have leukemia. Only about 10% of cancer patients have blood borne disease. So 90% of people in need of treatment require something other than the relatively effective leukemia therapies.

I realized I had to break from my lovely little cool scientific pursuits if I was really going to change the history of cancer medicine. What I wanted to do then was step up to the solid tumors of the world. The uterines and ovaries. The breasts. The colons, the lungs, the gastrics, the biliaries and pancreatics. All the diseases that kill people. When I did that, my lovely little delightful cool scientific opportunities fell apart.

Why? Well, first, you couldn't isolate a pure cancer cell to study DNA degradation, or whatever I was working on. You couldn't do flow cytometry on solids. You had to come up with different platforms. It became evident to me that cancer solid tumors were not cells but systems. Cancer in a solid tumor environment isn't a cell bouncing around in your bloodstream. It is a collection of cancer cells talking to one another. Talking to the stroma, talking to the cancer-associated fibroblasts, talking to the T-cells, talking to the B-cells, talking to the M-2 macrophages, and interacting within this microenvironment world.

When I tried to recreate blood borne tumors, by disaggregating my solid tumors down to single cells, and then studying them, it didn't predict much. So I thought, well maybe the cancer is more complicated than just the cell. Maybe it's the dysregulated system.

A very interesting investigation from Lawrence Livermore Lab, showcased an experiment that has never left my mind. The researcher took breast epithelial cell lines, and she placed them in growth media to grow them. If she introduced certain conditions, certain fibroblast conditions, and certain growth factors, she could make these benign cell lines grow into cancers. If she took another collection of these cells, and she grew them under other conditions, they became benign epithelial organs, like little microorganisms. So she could make cancer grow depending on the conditions of the growth media. She could grow cancers—or not—that had nothing to do with the DNA of the cell.

What we realized was we needed to study cancer systems, not cancer cells. So we developed technology to isolate three-dimensional Explants. So we went from hemes, which we still do, into solids, which we've done more in the last twenty years. And we developed a platform that allows us to study not cells, but micro Explants, three dimensional Explants. That's the principal model we now use. Cancer in the test tube that looks precisely like it does in your body.

Ann: In a nutshell, what can patients expect if they request services from the Nagourney Cancer Institute?

Dr. Nagourney: I have a very accommodating staff, who will do their best to help. We need to get a piece of tumor. If it's bloodborne, it's simple. We just draw blood. If it's a solid tumor, we would need to work with a surgeon, or people can visit us, and we will conduct the procedure here. We need about a cubic centimeter of viable tissue. A lima bean sized tissue sample, which is then transported by overnight courier. We arrange the courier. We arrange the whole deal. When we receive the sample, we begin our study. Results will be available about a week later. We are always glad to work with patients' doctors. If there are drugs or certain combinations that are of particular interest, we will always do our best to accommodate those interests whether they're single agents, targeted agents, metabolic inhibitors, or combinations. We will do everything within our power to provide the patient the most useful information. The service itself is about a week turnaround, and we need a little coordination so we can work with the surgeon or interventional radiologist or someone doing thoracentesis or paracentesis to obtain, and then transport, the sample. Mostly, we have to work with the people on site to ensure the process is done correctly.

Ann: You recommend, but do not provide, treatment...

Dr. Nagourney: That's not true. I do.

Ann: So you do provide actual treatment?

Dr. Nagourney: I do. I was just at the hospital, and I'll be returning once we're done. In my group, there are only two MDs. I generally only accept patients if no one else will treat them.

Ann: Do you maintain a list of practitioners you work with?

Dr. Nagourney: I tell patients that they need to understand that our role in this, at least at first pass, is to identify available treatments and combinations that are widely used. We pick the ones that are best. Their medical oncologist should be very familiar with the recommendation. For example, let's look at uterine cancer. What's the treatment? Well, most people give carboplatin and Taxol. There was a study done some years ago by Scottish investigators called the Scot Roc. It showed that in gynecologic malignancies, carboplatin plus Taxotere is equivalent on every level. For some patients, it's less toxic. We published that carboplatin or cisplatin plus gemcitabine is extremely effective. We have also been able to study carboplatin plus doxorubicin, so all of these regimens exist. It's not like I'm inventing them. They're out there. It's simply that individual doctors choose one over another, and his/her choice might be wrong for their patient.

They are doing a disservice to their patient by not using another, perfectly appropriate, available FDA approved combination. What we have here is another example of denialism. Doctors who don't want to use scientific evidence and instead would like to use their whims. What we say to patients is, "Look. We will do this study. We have expansive experience. If your doctor doesn't want to treat you, I will." That's my offer.

Ann: Thank you for clarifying that. It's good to know, and I'm sure people reading the book will be grateful to hear that. You've covered this to some extent, but what are your current theories about the etiology of cancer?

Dr. Nagourney: You had posed a couple of questions. One of them was about metabolism. I saw you were referencing Mark Lintern. I've read some of his material. The only thing that strikes me about this guy is he's a non-oncologist taking a jaundiced eye look at the absurdity of modern oncology and saying, "Gee, this emperor has no clothes."

I don't find his work compelling or scientifically interesting. None of the things he says are original, but let's face it. Cancer medicine has gone down one, solitary direction: the gene profile, cancer as a genetic disorder. I've been describing that as a falsehood for three decades. Cancer is far more than simply genes. It's biosystematic approaches. If there's any question about this, you have to understand that LeRoy Hood, who invented the gene sequencer, left genomics for systems biology twenty-five years ago. If the guy who developed the ability to sequence genes figured that theory about cancer was inadequate, why is everyone else continuing to cling to it?

When you asked me about the origins of cancer, they're distinctly different from what people think. Today, if you ask most medical oncologists and scientists, what causes cancer, they'll tell you it's a genetic disorder. There's a mutation, it leads to a certain adaptation, and then there's another mutation. So that's the mutational theory.

I don't think that's correct at all. Cancer is a cell that needs something. Within our trillions of cells within our bodies, we are continually producing more cells. Your breasts, your uterus, your prostate, your stomach lining are all reproducing. A cell in the middle of your body is missing something. It's not getting enough blood supply or oxygen or nutrients or glutamine, growth factor, estrogen, etc. The cell looks around and says, "Gee, I'm going to die. I can't get my _____." So the cell says maybe there's a way around this blockade. It reaches deep into its pocket and comes up with a gene. That gene may be a normal gene, but the cell will use it abnormally. Or it might be an abnormal gene that's adapted to the cell. The cell selects genetic elements toward its greater good. It applies what it has at its disposal. We've got this whole thing backward thinking it's a mutation that causes the cell to become cancerous when it's actually the cell that drives the mutation.

That's why many of the mutational findings of cancer are shared. All the cancer cells in the world are going to use RAS or P53 or PIK3CA or something because they're all trying to get the nutrients and substances they need to survive. Cancer is a disease of cells trying to stay alive and a body trying to kill them.

Ann: How do you feel about the Warburg effect?

Dr. Nagourney: Otto Warburg was unequivocally brilliant. He was a Nobel laureate. He described metabolic abnormalities of cancer cells that are fundamental to our modern understanding of tumor biology. But to quote Otto Warburg, like Jack Horner, who stuck in his thumb and pulled out a plum, is naïve. Warburg's work indicated that cancer is a disease of cells that were trying to survive using energy. That is fundamental to our modern understanding of cancer. And yes, if you go to a cancer research meeting today, you will not be able to go to a lecture where someone doesn't start off by saying, "Otto Warburg..."

Let me tell you something about cancer. Cancer medicine will clearly clock around to metabolic studies. But the trouble with all of this is cancer is like the weather: everybody talks about it, but no one does anything. We are doing something. I started out as a chemist. I knew from the get-go that cancer was a metabolic disorder. I understood cancer was to be discerned biochemically. There was no chance on God's green earth we were going to come up with a gene answer.

And we haven't. So, I realized we were going to have to get down to the nitty gritty of the biochemistry and the enzymology that characterized the great breakthroughs of medicine until the 1950s when we had the misfortune of discovering the structure of DNA in 1953. That launched a thousand ships in the wrong direction. Everyone said, "Oho. We've got the DNA structure. We can now cure cancer."

I am still waiting. Seventy years and counting.

People who took their ideas, including LeRoy Hood, who thought since it was a gene story, let's dig down into the genes, were destined to fail. Determined to figure it out, he invented the gene sequencer. He was basically the father of modern genomics, and he left it. My late friend Cary Mulis invented PCR. He thought it was a diagnostic technique. He never thought that gene sequencing and gene analysis were ever going to cure cancer. He got a Nobel prize in 1992. The smart guys left this dumb idea a long time ago.

Ann: This is interesting and validating for me. So thank you for that. Are you familiar with Travera?

Dr. Nagourney: They are one of many companies that have again stuck their thumb into a pie, pulled out a plum, and said what a good boy am I. They are all part of the institutional denialism that had no interest in human tissue primary cultures for decades, who thought it was a bunch of hooey. Suddenly, they realize it works.

Now they're going to invent it. These are modern millennials who think they invented everything and have failed to offer any credit to those of us who actually did. Travera's technique was developed by MIT. It's a cellular mass technique. So what do they do? They isolate cancer cells and put them into a very accurate measure to see if the cells, when exposed to certain drugs, will begin to suffer injury that leads to death. We did that sort of stuff with CLL twenty-five years ago. Within four to eight hours, we could see evidence of programmed cell death developing as DNA degradation yielded to activated apoptosis. We know that cells commit to death when exposed to drugs. The question for a company like Travera is does the measure of a single cell injured by drugs predict outcome?

So you go to their website and you see what their references are. They have case reports of a patient who got better when they picked the drug. If they're going to base their work on that, they should buy lottery tickets because one in nine million wins there too.

I had this conversation with Travera. I was asked to give a symposium about prostate cancer, and these guys came along and said, "Oh, we're doing this, too."

I wrote back to them and asked if they'd done the fundamental work that makes this effective. For example, had they applied this technology—at MIT or not—to determine if the drugs we know work, will work in their test? For example, ARAC works in leukemia. It does not work in lung cancer. Cisplatin works in lung cancer. It does not work in leukemia. Have they taken the trouble to show that they can reproduce history? Have they taken the trouble to do retrospective analysis on people who've received different treatments where they had the opportunity to test them to see if their outcomes were predictable. Have they done prospective trials to take forward with their test to see if they are accurately identifying patients who will benefit from their interventions?

If you go back through the history of this field, you'll see that people like Deborah Schragg and the Blue Cross/Blue Shield Technology Assessment Group, decided to trash it. We had an up and back battle, including the Wall Street Journal, where they were wrong, and we were right. We editorialized in the JCO, and they wrote another paper and admitted they'd been wrong and that the field had merit, but it still wasn't mature. The point is what they were criticizing: cancer as a metabolic disease. Many very good investigators did extensive work in this field. Andrew Bosanquett from England was brilliant. Peter Twentyman, also from England, was brilliant. These guys were doing great work thirty years ago, and they were never credited for it. That's a great tragedy.

However, now MIT or Harvard comes along, and suddenly, you don't need to prove it anymore. It's no longer necessary to prove that this works. It's just a really good idea that everyone should do. A joke I heard a few years ago from one of my colleagues at UC Irvine where I teach was that a guy came up with a breakthrough drug that when administered to mice with cancer cured every mouse. He said, "My goodness, that's brilliant. I've never seen data like this. When do we get to apply this mouse data to people?"

The answer was, "Oh, that's easy. When the mouse data is generated at Harvard."

Travera and others like them have failed to reference the work that came before. People have been doing incredible work these last thirty or forty years. I'm not taking credit for it. There have been many exceptional investigators, who get no credit for fighting uphill against people like these guys. They're the same ones who made it tough to get papers published and grants funded.

Ann: The encouraging part to me about Travera—win, lose, or draw—is it's accepted by mainstream oncology. My limited experience with them was if you don't do it cookie-cutter, by the book, they don't want to talk to you.

Dr. Nagourney: Imagine if mainstream oncology accepts Travera and others like them, and it doesn't work. My greatest fear here is these people will come up with these great ideas, but their execution will be lacking. Travera is not the only one. There's one in Seattle, another in Vanderbilt. They're selling similar products. Imagine if Travera designs a study, and it fails. Do you know what that does to the field?

There's plenty of room for good laboratories, but they have no idea if their technology is good, they're just selling it.

Ann: This is all grist for the mill. In one of the chapters in the book, I got permission from John Horgan, a well-known science writer, to reproduce an article he'd written in 2019 about the cancer industry and hype versus reality. He builds a pretty solid argument that not only are we not winning the war against cancer, but we've actually lost ground. I'm just encouraged whenever anything that's a breath of fresh air comes along.

Dr. Nagourney: If it's a breath of fresh air that's contaminated, it's not so refreshing.

Ann: You're absolutely right.

Dr. Nagourney: So many of the large cancer centers have now jumped on this bandwagon. Dana Farber. Sloan Kettering is attempting this using propagated organoids. These guys are all banking on the concept working. If it doesn't. If David Tuveson's trial at Sloan Kettering is not successful, for the wrong reasons, it will damage the field. The real work in this field is what's called three-dimensional Explants.

That's the difference. Three dimensional Explants that recreate the microenvironmental conditions of the cancer that lives in your body. If these guys at MIT take one cell out and isolate it from its stroma and its fibroblasts and its T and B cells, and its macrophages, they then create a highly artificial environment. Exposing cells to it may, or may not, be predicting outcomes. If it does not work. If they do clinical trials someday, and it does not work, the field will be damaged.

The reason I'm fearful of that is I think they're doing it wrong. If it doesn't work, they will say the field is bad rather than their techniques.

Ann: We can adopt a watch and wait and hope for the best.

Dr. Nagourney: The people who quote Otto Warburg are not particularly sophisticated when it comes to what he said. I realized many years ago that cancer was more likely to be a biochemical disturbance than a genetic disorder. It certainly isn't a genetic disorder. I've never varied from that in over thirty years. However, no one outside of quoting Warburg, is doing anything valid except us.

We built a mass spectrometry laboratory in my clinic. We built a lab to measure the metabolism of cancer, and we have published a few papers that are so stunning they represent landmark changes in the way we think. I can quote one for you. It's in Gynecologic Oncology from 2021. You can look it up. We used plasma metabolism, the study of how cells make and use energy, to predict survival in ovarian cancer. It is a stunning example of what we can do in the future. We also reported last year, in the American Association of Cancer Research, that if you take cells and place them into a tissue culture media, those cancer cells in their own little world are using and making energy. They generate patterns of metabolism that can be measured via metabolites. So we examined the media from the cancer cells. They were sitting quietly in their media in the incubator without any drugs, just cancer cells and tissue media. We studied the media to see what the cancer cells were making and using. Building on that, we could predict who was going to survive ovarian cancer four days after diagnosis.

Ann: That's impressive.

Dr. Nagourney: I do a lot of basic research. Our latest paper is on P53, a regulator for cell survival. That's not particularly germane to what we're talking about. What you're interested in is you're looking for alternative conceptual frameworks for cancer biology. Survival curves are predicated not on DNA, but on what the patients' tumors are using for energy. It represents a fundamental change in the direction of cancer medicine.

Ann: You've given me a lot of your time here. Do you have words of hope for those of us who, for one reason or another, ended up with cancer, especially stage four?

Dr. Nagourney: Metastatic disease constitutes the majority of pancreatic cancer patients, a substantial plurality of colon cancer patients, and a substantial plurality of gastric cancer. According to a study just published by the JNCI, there has been virtually no change in survival for metastatic disease. Despite the great clamor surrounding targeted agents, the average improvement in survival with targeted agents has been in the range of three months. These are drugs that cost $12,000 a month, so we are not winning this war.

When you ask me what I would say, there is no one more interested in saving your life than you. You must become your own champion and challenge the dogma that has led to the dismal outcomes in modern oncology. What we have are people who are afraid to step outside the confines of standards and community standards to help their patients. Doctors would rather lose a patient than save them using something that might draw criticism. Doctors have lost touch with what they're doing. Doctors should be saviors, not trialists.

Ann: When I taught at the family medicine residency, residents were more than willing to research things and do things outside recognized standard of care. Something happens between being trained in one subspecialty versus being trained in another.

Dr. Nagourney: I'll tell you what happens. Evidence-based medicine. It is the modern religion. It's the cudgel used by relatively unimaginative doctors to prevent anyone from doing anything differently from what they're doing. If you really drill down to the merits of evidence-based medicine, it falls apart immediately. For example, if a colleague asks, "Where's the evidence?" I will ask him what color shirt he's wearing. When he says blue, I'll ask if there is a control group that was tested to prove that the color of your shirt is blue.

Has anyone ever done a clinical trial to prove appendectomies save lives? Of course not. Has anyone ever done a clinical trial to prove parachutes save lives? Of course not. This premise that everything has to be proven is an utter fallacy.

But they use it as a cudgel. If you read the truest meaning of evidence-based medicine, it is to use evidence. Where high level evidence exists, you apply it. Where low level evidence exists, and circumstances haven't leant themselves to higher levels, you use that. Evidence-based medicine is completely abused by the medical community. When a primary care doctor finds a problem, he doesn't usually refer to the literature, he simply fixes it. He doesn't ask if there's a clinical trial to corroborate that suturing a wound helps people, he just does it.

As you move up the ladder where survival curves are measured in calipers, outcomes become meaningless. New drugs might give us three months of survival. A published clinical trial of a cancer agent added ten days to lifespans of pancreatic cancer patients. The FDA approved it. This is why people like Lintern look at medical oncology and say, "This is ridiculous." If he was dependent on peer-reviewed journals or Federal grants, he wouldn't be saying these things. Because he's not an MD, it offers him latitude.

Everyone is cowed into not telling the truth. It's a big problem.

Ann: That's mildly depressing. And being a patient stuck in that system is even more depressing.

Dr. Nagourney: Remember, we still live in a free country, so then you can make decisions if you're not happy with the dismal survival curves they show you. You can tell your oncologist, "That's not good enough." This is the power this book has to bring to the table as it encourages patients to not accept dogma, if that dogma turns them into a statistic rather than a person. Doctors have forgotten who they work for.

They work for the patient, and they're supposed to do everything in their power to get their patients better. That's why I do what I do. My relationship is with my patients, not with my academic community. I don't care anymore. I'm interested in patient outcomes. That's what drives me. It's an uphill battle to do what I do. It's not easy. It's not rewarding. It's not financially rewarding, but it is extraordinarily rewarding when patients survive.

Most of the patients who come to me are untreatable. They have no options, and fully half of them get better.

Ann: That's incredibly impressive. Thank you so much for your generosity in making time for me and being willing to sit for an interview for *Alive, Surviving Modern Oncology*. I'm certain readers will appreciate your candor and the breadth of your experience and wisdom.

Dr. Nagourney: To close, I'm hoping that some of the work we're doing, and others, will allow us to identify drugs that are selectively toxic to cancer cells that are using abnormal metabolism to stay alive. So, that's hopefully the future. That's why we're doing what we're doing.

What Causes Cancer Anyway?

After Dr. Nagourney's elegant and succinct description regarding the etiology of cancer, I debated deleting this chapter. Still, it was already written and it delves into some history that is quite intriguing. We've skirted around "right" answers to this question but have been sidetracked many, many times.

Cancer is a complex, multifaceted problem. I am neither scientist nor medical doctor. I certainly don't have a definitive answer to this question, but until we can home in on what something is, there won't be concordance about how to treat it.

Indulge me in a bit of historical retrospective. It's easier to appreciate where we are now if we know where we began. Much of the information in the following pages came from an article in the New York Times Magazine by Sam Apple, written in 2016. He kindly provided permission to reproduce a few paragraphs.

For a long while, cancer was viewed as a genetic disease involving nuclear mutations in oncogenesis and tumor suppressor genes. Certain mutations, like BRCA 1 and 2, were supposed to predispose people to more intractable cancers.

Lynch syndrome is an inherited genetic disorder linked to an increased risk of developing cancer, often at a younger age in life—especially colorectal cancer, and, for women, endometrial cancer. While those are the most common types of cancer associated with the disorder, it is also tied to a greater lifetime risk of other types of cancer, including stomach, small intestine, liver, ovarian, upper urinary tract, gallbladder ducts, brain, and skin.

Not everyone with BRCA will develop cancer. Likewise, not everyone with Lynch syndrome will, either. The risk with Lynch depends, in part, on which of the five Lynch syndrome-responsible genes has the inherited genetic defect and the types of cancer that have been diagnosed throughout a family's medical history. For perspective, Lynch syndrome accounts for about 3 percent of colorectal cancers and 2 percent of endometrial cancers.

Lynch syndrome is one of the few "Tier 1 genomic conditions" included in a list that the Centers for Disease Control and Prevention (CDC) promotes as genetic conditions that can and should be monitored to improve or prevent health issues. The earlier a person is aware of the condition, the more opportunities exist to take preventative actions to reduce the risk of developing cancer.

Despite the pervasive evidence of a genetic basis for Lynch, many inconsistencies plague the somatic mutation theory. The most salient includes many large population-based studies that compared tens of thousands of people with similar genetic patterning. Some got cancer; others didn't. If a somatic mutation theory were the true underpinning of cancer, everyone with a certain mutation would end up cancer. In most cases, it's a mere handful.

Emerging evidence suggests cancer is a mitochondrial metabolic disease, according to the original theory of Otto Warburg.

Dr. Warburg, a German physiologist, medical doctor, and Nobel laureate, was the first to promote the idea of treating cancer by starving its source of energy. Since many cancers utilize glucose-driven pathways, avoiding sugar was part of his protocol.

No one took his ideas seriously until this past decade when cutting edge books like, *How to Starve Cancer Without Starving Yourself* by McLelland and *The Metabolic Theory of Cancer* by Winters became popular.

Many cancer patients who adhered to these principles not only survived but thrived.

The following is from Sam Apple's article.

"Modern cancer research began somewhat improbably with the sea urchin. In the first decade of the 20th century, the

German biologist Theodor Boveri fertilized sea urchin eggs with two sperm rather than one. The result was some of the cells ended up with the wrong number of chromosomes and failed to develop properly. This was before modern genetics, but cancer cells, like deformed sea urchin cells, had abnormal chromosomes. Boveri surmised cancer had something to do with chromosomes."

"Today Boveri is celebrated for discovering the origins of cancer, but Otto Warburg was studying sea urchin eggs around the same time. His research was hailed as a major breakthrough in our understanding of cancer. For whatever reason, in the following decades, his work would largely disappear."

"Unlike Boveri, Warburg wasn't interested in the chromosomes of sea urchin eggs. Rather, he was focused on energy, specifically on how the eggs fueled their growth. By the time Warburg turned his attention from sea urchin cells to the cells of a rat tumor, in 1923, he knew that sea urchin eggs increased their oxygen consumption significantly as they grew, so he expected to see a similar need for extra oxygen in the rat tumor. Instead, the cancer cells fueled their growth by swallowing up enormous amounts of glucose (blood sugar) and breaking it down without oxygen. The result made no sense. Oxygen-fueled reactions are a much more efficient way of turning food into energy, and there was plenty of oxygen available for the cancer cells to use. When Warburg tested additional tumors, including ones from humans, he found the same effect every time."

"Cancer cells were ravenous for glucose."

"This discovery, later named the Warburg effect, is estimated to occur in up to 80 percent of cancers. It is so fundamental to most cancers that a positron emission tomography (PET) scan, which has emerged as an important tool in the staging and diagnosis of cancer, works simply by revealing the places in the body where cells are consuming extra glucose. In many cases, the more glucose a tumor consumes, the worse a patient's prognosis."

As a passing note, PET scans utilize an obscene amount of radiation. Cancer patients might not want to have very many of them because radiation is far from benign and can cause the growth of different cancers years down the line.

"Following this breakthrough, Warburg became convinced the Warburg effect occurred because cells were unable to use oxygen properly and that this damaged respiration was, in effect, the starting point of cancer. Well into the 1950s, this theory—which Warburg believed in until his death in 1970 but never proved—remained an important subject of debate within the field."

"Unfortunately, more quickly than anyone could have anticipated, the debate ended. In 1953, James Watson and Francis Crick pieced together the structure of the DNA molecule and set the stage for the triumph of molecular biology's gene-centered approach to cancer. In the following decades, scientists came to regard cancer as a disease governed by mutated genes, which drove cells into a state of relentless division and proliferation. The metabolic catalysts that Warburg spent his career analyzing began to be referred to as "housekeeping enzymes"—necessary to keep a cell going but largely irrelevant to the deeper story of cancer."

"Boston College biologist, Thomas Seyfried, characterized the shift to molecular biology as a stampede. Warburg was dropped like yesterday's news. There was every reason to think Warburg would remain at best a footnote in the history of cancer research, but over the past decade, and the past five years in particular, something unexpected happened: Those housekeeping enzymes have again become one of the most promising areas of cancer research. Scientists now wonder if metabolism could prove to be the long-sought "Achilles' heel" of cancer, a common weak point in a disease that manifests itself in so many different forms."

"There are typically many mutations in a single cancer. But there are a limited number of ways bodies can produce energy and support rapid growth. Cancer cells rely on these fuels in a way healthy cells don't. The hope of scientists at the forefront of the Warburg revival is that they will be able to slow—or even stop—tumors by disrupting one or more of the many chemical reactions a cell uses to proliferate. In the process, they will starve cancer cells of the nutrients they desperately need to grow."

"Even James Watson, one of the fathers of molecular biology, is convinced targeting metabolism is a more promising avenue in current cancer research than gene-centered approaches. A direct quote from Watson at the age of 88 is: 'Locating the genes that cause cancer has been remarkably unhelpful. The belief that sequencing your DNA is going to extend your life is a cruel illusion.'"

"Back to Warburg. He appreciated that a tumor's dependence upon a steady flow of nutrients might eventually prove to be its fatal weakness. Long after his initial discovery of the Warburg effect, he continued to research the enzymes involved in fermentation and to explore the possibility of blocking the process in cancer cells. The challenge Warburg faced then is the same one metabolism researchers face today: Cancer is an incredibly persistent foe. Blocking one metabolic pathway has been shown to slow down and even stop tumor growth in some cases, but tumors tend to find another way. If you block glucose, they use glutamine, another primary fuel. If you block glucose and glutamine, they might be able to use fatty acids."

One of the obvious downsides of trying to block every pathway is a patient will eventually starve themselves in the process. Staying one step ahead of cancer is important, but you have to do it judiciously.

"Given Warburg's own story of historical neglect, it's fitting that what may turn out to be one of the most promising cancer metabolism drugs has been sitting in plain sight for decades. That drug, metformin, is already widely prescribed to decrease blood glucose in diabetics."

Today, it's commonly used to treat—or prevent—cancer. It's a frequent integrative approach. Most standard of care oncologists will not write you a prescription for this "can't hurt, might help," drug.

Integrative oncologists, however, will.

"Because metformin can influence a number of metabolic pathways, the precise mechanism by which it achieves its anticancer effects remains a source of debate. But the results of numerous epidemiological studies have been striking. Diabetics taking metformin seem to be significantly less likely to develop cancer than diabetics who don't. Those on metformin are significantly less likely to die from cancer if they do contract it."

"Near the end of his life, Warburg grew obsessed with his diet. He believed most cancer was preventable and thought chemicals added to food and used in agriculture could cause tumors by interfering with respiration. He stopped eating bread unless it was baked in his own home. He would drink milk only if it came from a special herd of cows and used a centrifuge at his lab to make his cream and butter."

"Warburg's personal diet is unlikely to become a path to prevention. But the Warburg revival has allowed researchers to develop a hypothesis for how diets linked to our obesity and diabetes epidemics—specifically, sugar-heavy diets that can result in permanently elevated levels of the hormone insulin—may also be driving cells to the Warburg effect and cancer."

"The insulin hypothesis can be traced to the research of Lewis Cantley, the director of the Meyer Cancer Center at Weill Cornell Medical College. In the 1980s, Cantley discovered how insulin, which is released by the pancreas and tells cells to take up glucose, influences what happens inside a cell. Cantley now refers to insulin and a closely related hormone, IGF-1 (insulinlike growth factor 1), as "the champion" activators of metabolic proteins linked to cancer. He's beginning to see evidence, he says, that in some cases, 'it really is insulin itself that's getting the tumor started.'"

"One way to think about the Warburg effect is as the insulin, or IGF-1, signaling pathway "gone awry—its cells behaving as though insulin were telling it to take up glucose all the time and to grow." Cantley, who avoids eating sugar as much as he can, is currently studying the effects of diet on mice that have the mutations commonly found in colorectal and other cancers. He says that the effects of a sugary diet on colorectal, breast and other cancer models 'looks very impressive' and "'scary.'"

"Elevated insulin is also strongly associated with obesity, which is expected to overtake smoking as the leading cause of preventable cancer. Cancers linked to obesity and diabetes have more receptors for insulin and IGF-1, and people with defective IGF-1 receptors appear to be nearly immune to cancer. Retrospective studies, which look back at patient histories, suggest many people who develop colorectal, pancreatic, or breast cancer have elevated insulin levels before diagnosis. It's perhaps not entirely surprising, then, that when researchers want to grow breast-cancer cells in the lab, they add insulin to the tissue culture."

"When they remove the insulin, the cancer cells die."

"During Warburg's lifetime, insulin's effects on metabolic pathways were even less well understood. It's highly unlikely he would have considered the possibility that anything other than damaged respiration could cause cancer. He died sure that he was right about the disease. A framed quote from Max Planck hung above his desk."

"It read, 'A new scientific truth does not triumph by convincing its opponents and making them see the light, but rather because its opponents eventually die.'"

I hope this segue into the history of cancer was interesting to read. Again, many thanks to Sam Apple for his article in the New York Times magazine. I borrowed heavily from it with a few parenthetical comments added. If you want to know more about Otto Warburg, take a look at Sam's book titled, *Ravenous*. It's a fascinating read, and it's listed in the resource section.

An upshot of my research is that diet and supplements are essential to address both prevention and treatment of cancer. To keep on eating sugar and sugary foods is foolhardy, no matter what MDs, most of whom received minimal training in nutrition in medical school, might tell you.

Again, do your own research.

Continuing with a departure from the somatic mutation theory, below are wheels depicting the hallmarks of cancer as described by Hanahan and Weinberg's 2011 paper, updated in 2022. On the left are the original ten hallmarks of cancer. The righthand wheel creates an argument to add four more to the mix. If you'd like to read the full article, here's the link.

https://aacrjournals.org/cancerdiscovery/article/12/1/31/675608/Hallmarks-of-Cancer-New-DimensionsHallmarks-of (for those reading the paperback)

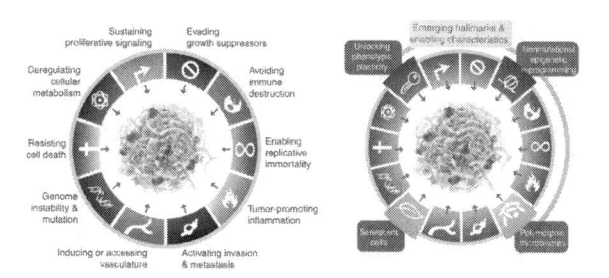

There's one more topic I'd like to broach before we leave this chapter. One of the contributors to *Alive* brought a paper by Mark Lintern to my attention. Mr. Lintern spent the last eight years working on his own theories about cancer. He favors a cell suppression approach. A transcript of one of his paper, "Cancer Through Another Lens," is included in the resource section at the back of this book. He has also written a book, *The Cancer Resolution*, on the topic. Podcasts of his research are available through Say Yes to Life on YouTube.

Paraphrasing, Lintern asks the question: what if the abnormal behavior of a cancer cell is not a result of malfunction, but of suppression, where an external factor foreign to the cell influences cell death and growth mechanisms, leaving the cell no longer in full control?

Multiple studies confirm that, upon infection, pathogens instigate the Warburg effect. It could be viewed as a natural anti-infection response.

Here, hiding in plain sight, is a known cause for the Warburg effect, ignored until now due to the common assertion that cancer results from faulty cell machinery. While the notion of cancer resulting from infection is not new, this cell suppression concept is unique and has yet to be explored by scientists. Currently, around 20 percent of cancers are associated with infection, but not in a suppressive capacity; rather, micro-organisms are thought to damage the cell leading to malfunction. It is this malfunctioning cell machinery that is ultimately thought to be driving the disease, rather than the micro-organism per se.

Lintern proposes that the suppressive nature of the pathogen and its control over specific cellular functions, such as cell death and cell growth mechanisms, drives the disease, not the random damage inflicted by infection or carcinogens.

This would explain why anti-parasitic drugs like Mebendazole, Fenbendazole, and Ivermectin are useful as adjunctive treatments. Doxycycline falls into the same camp. It also explains why measures of inflammation don't bode well for survival.

One bottom line is we do not yet know what causes cancer with any degree of certainty. We are getting closer, though. Once we can answer this very important question, our current treatments will go the way of the Dodo bird in favor of less toxic, more humane interventions that produce better outcomes because they are specifically targeted to each person's individual physiology.

For those so inclined, here's a link (see below for the full link for those reading a paperback copy) to a recent intriguing podcast from Jason Fung, M.D. and Sanjay Juneja, M.D., discussing ideas about how cancer behaves more like a single-celled organism than one belonging within a human body where cooperation among parts is essential for survival. Drs. Fung and Juneja build a case for minimal amounts of chemotherapy—as opposed to the maximum tolerated dose—since cancer cells develop resistance. They also expand on the fact that a kernel of cancer is in every one of our cells and discuss what pushes evolutionary changes that drive the mutations that turn into cancer. Frankly, I found it intriguing.

I will expand on the relatively new field of integrative oncology in another chapter at the end of this book.

Let's look at a couple of survivor stories before my personal story unfolds.

Link to Dr. Fung's podcast:

https://podcasts.apple.com/us/podcast/target-cancer-podcast/id1593087681?i=1000617826771

Karen's Story

I am 73 - I have fibromyalgia (I was hit by a drunk driver at age 20 and had really bad whiplash.) the Fibro started in my early 40s, but I have always had trouble with my neck since the accident.

In 2000 I was diagnosed with a muli-nodular goiter of the thyroid (non-cancerous). I took thyroid medicine for 12 years to suppress it but it continued to get larger. In 2012 I had my thyroid removed (still non-cancerous), and now I take thyroid replacement medicine.

There is a lot of info about trauma causing cancer. My childhood was definitely non-traumatic! I was very lucky to grow up in a loving normal family!

My first physical (and some mental) trauma was when I got hit by the drunk driver! From 1998 to 2002, we lived in NYC. **9/11 BLEW MY MIND** in so many ways! By the summer of 2002, I was having ovarian pain. A CT showed what they thought was a teratoma. We were moving back to Atlanta, so I sought treatment there. As a side note, when I began looking for work after our move from Atlanta to NYC, the employment agency wanted me to interview in the Twin Towers and my instantaneous reply was, "Oh no, they bombed it once and I think they will try again!"

She told me I would make $10K-$20K more and cut my commute by 20 or 30 minutes but that did not dissuade me. I do believe in guardian angels! I also missed a train in Italy that was bombed! So I believe in listening to my guardian angels/gut instincts!

In August of 2002 I had a laparoscopic hysterectomy because of the suspected teratoma on my ovary and a prolapsing uterus. They wound up removing both ovaries along with my uterus. The doctor said one ovary was basically dead and the other was over producing hormones. That would explain the hot flashes I had been having.

However, the doctor **never** told me that I had **granulosa cell tumor ovarian cancer (a very rare form of ovarian cancer - only about 4-5% of all ovarian cancers)**! In my post-op appointment, I asked him, "Was it a teratoma?" He said no. I said, "So what was it? Was it cancer?" He told me no it wasn't cancer and just come back for yearly PAP smears!! I did not find out that I had cancer until 14 years later when I had a recurrence. I went to the ER in severe pain in my right shoulder in Dec. 2015. They ran the usual heart tests, then did a CT which came back with a suspected hemangioma on my liver.

I had requested my medical records from the doctor who did my hysterectomy because we had moved and I needed a new doctor. I went to see a liver specialist at Emory and when he saw my records, he sent me to a gynecologist!

Emory is a teaching hospital, so the first person to see was an intern in training and she said to me, "So, have you had chemo?" I said, "No, why would I have had chemo?" She said, "Because you have ovarian cancer."

You could have knocked me over with a feather! I was briefly hysterical! The gynecologist scheduled me for a colonoscopy and a PET scan. The PET lit up a baseball size tumor in my lower pelvic basin. Then they did a biopsy which revealed that the pelvic tumor was **granulosa cell tumor ovarian cancer (GCT)**.

The suspicious area on my liver came back hemangioma (this later turned out to be wrong). The Emory doctor wanted to schedule me for surgery to remove the pelvic tumor but she wanted permission to give me a colostomy or ileostomy if she felt it was necessary.

I refused.

I refuse to live my life with poop bags hanging off of me, and I felt her approach was excessive! She then suggested chemo to shrink the tumor, but I had already done enough research to know that chemo was not the recommended course of treatment for GCT. The first line of treatment is surgery with hormone suppression drugs afterward.

So, I ran!

I found a gynecological oncologist at Northeast Georgia Health System, who agreed with me that chemo is not the recommended treatment, and he agreed not to do a colostomy or ileostomy (I also write this on my surgical permission forms and initial it). I had a successful surgery in March of 2016 to remove the pelvic tumor. He also took off the top 1/4 of my vagina with my cervix which left me very vexed as that was never discussed!

Recovery was the usual 10-12 weeks. Afterwards I contacted a malpractice attorney to sue the fist doctor who did my hysterectomy but did not tell me my diagnosis. Because so much time had gone by, my attorney said it would be difficult to win in court, so I wound up settling out of court. I did not get very much, but it gave me the satisfaction of proving the doctor was negligent.

It turned out he was being sued by a few others as well!

I continued to have bloodwork and MRIs every 6 months (sometimes I opted for ultrasounds instead just to give my body a break from the chemicals.) By 2019, the "hemangioma" was larger, so I went back to the liver doctor at Emory (who probably saved my life by sending me to a gynecologist) to see what to do.

He wanted to take out 2/3 of my liver! Because Emory is so far from where I live, I asked for the name of a doctor who was closer to me. This very elderly doctor also wanted to take out 2/3 of my liver and gave me a printout of all the risks and complications. Once again, I listened to my guardian angel and felt that this approach could kill me and was way too risky.

I did some more research and found an amazing liver and pancreas specialist at Northside Hospital in Atlanta. He gave my CT images to his radiologist to look at, and they both agreed that the "hemangioma" was likely GCT but that it was not IN my liver but trapped between my liver and diaphragm. I also had some small spots in my lower pelvic region.

In Feb. of 2020, I had surgery with the liver doctor and the gynecological doctor and was declared NED afterward. The liver doctor saved my life. The pathology report came back that the "hemangioma" was actually GCT and that the Emory biopsy was wrong!

I will never return to Emory!!

Then Covid happened! I am sure that my follow up care was not up to par, but I was still getting bloodwork and ultrasounds, just not as often. In April of 2022, a CT showed new but tiny tumors in my lower pelvic region. In July I got Covid (stayed home and recovered without hospitalization).

By September, the CT showed the tumors had doubled in size! My gut tells me this was because of Covid (I did not get the vaccine.) Because my surgeon from 2016 was being sued for malpractice, I started looking for a new doctor! I found one at a Northside facility closer to me, and my liver doctor from 2020 said he was an excellent surgeon.

In Jan 2023 I had my 3rd open abdomen surgery! They successfully removed two tumors but left me with two inoperable tumors - one next to my sigmoid colon and one near my iliac chain. My surgeon referred me to an oncologist. I am taking 2.5 mg of Letrozole daily and 7.5 mg monthly injection of Eligard - both hormone suppressors - side effects are general aches, minor light headedness, fatigue, tingling in lower legs and feet, and itchy bumps on upper back. After 2 shots, my InhibinB (best cancer marker for me) has dropped 670 points and the largest tumor shrank about 40%, so I am hopeful! I am trying to get PEF ablation (pulsed electric frequency) of the tumors at Duke.

I found out about PEF ablation from Dr. Jason Williams. It is a newer form of ablation with no thermal effect so there is less risk of damage to surrounding tissues. Because of the location of my tumors, this is really important! PEF ablation causes the outer "shell" of the tumor to become "porous" so that the immune system can see it. It also causes the abscopal effect, meaning that all the tumors respond, not just the ablated one! I am very hopeful! Dr. Williams and the Mayo Clinic in Jacksonville say it is definitely low risk and worth trying. I am lucky that I have no other health problems, except for the Fibro which I have had for so long that it is mostly background noise.

Lessons learned: Get copies of all your lab, surgery and pathology reports and **READ** them! Do not just rely on the doctor's word! That is what bit me in the butt in 2002! When I finally read the pathology report, it clearly said that I had GCT and that I should be followed closely! I was furious!

Such disregard and incompetence!

Do your research and join Facebook support groups, especially those specific to you type of cancer. I joined GCT Survivor Sisters, GCT Survivor Sister Holistic and GCT Warriors. I also joined Always Hope Cancer Protocol Support

Group and Healing Cancer Study Support Group. All these groups have TONS of helpful info! It is so important to be aware of what other rare GCT cancer patients are going through, what to avoid, and what they are doing to heal! It is also important to do your own research - http://www.targetedonc.com, NCBI, NIH, Drugs.com (check side effects and counterindications of your drugs), AACRJOURNALS, Pubmed, New England Journal of Medicine, Science Direct, clinical trials.gov ... so many good sources, sometimes overwhelming!

Greg's Story

... or ...

Cancer in 10 "Easy" Steps

① <u>Prepare for Life</u>

I arrived to the moment of my diagnosis 59 years of age, healthy and strong both mentally and physically with none of the usual ailments or comorbidities that typically accompany advanced middle age like hypertension, diabetes, high cholesterol, obesity, etc, etc.

Being able to focus on *just one problem* was a **great** blessing.

I credit maintaining a usually healthy omnivorous diet of fresh clean whole foods & pursuing sports ... ultra-trail running and mountaineering tied with a yoga practice.

These hobbies developed a mentality for discipline and perseverance in tackling big challenges. They also supported the robust energy I needed in my work as an entrepreneur in China.

Bad habits? Absolutely! Enjoying alcohol and the occasional cigars not to mention exposure to environmental toxins for which China is so famous.

Certainly not helpful ... but never particularly flagged by regular insurance company health checkups, either.

<u>Recommendation</u> ... always strive to improve/strengthen yourself mentally and physically. Not only to just "live your best life" but also, should tragedy strike, to be in better shape to weather it.

② <u>Self Awareness</u>

I felt an unusual pin prick sensation at the back of my throat. With a mirror, I could see the left side was different from the right. Obviously, I had a problem.

<u>Recommendation</u> ... pain is like a warning light on the dashboard. Ignore it at your peril.

③ <u>Timely Action</u>

I discussed it with my wife that same night over dinner and made an appointment for the next day to see an ENT physician at a top hospital with the equipment to make a conclusive diagnosis.

In 45 minutes the ENT physician had completed his observation, CT scan & biopsy. A few days later, the lab results confirmed the bad news.

HNSCC - (head and neck squamous cell carcinoma)

Local = left tonsil

Regional = left lymph nodes 2 level II, ½ level III, suspected involvement of back tongue left side and right-side neck lymph nodes.

Malignant, Stage IV

When your doctor tells you this, it's like walking through a portal to an alternate universe from where you can never return ... completely surreal.

<u>Recommendation</u> ... Never procrastinate. Problems only become worse with time and handling sooner is almost always easier. A well-defined problem can be handled far more efficiently and thoroughly.

④ <u>Self Education</u>

Diagnosis well in hand (or so I thought), I was able to put my attention to learning all about it through on-line research and discussions with top oncologists in Hong Kong and around the world.

Within a week, I discovered my ENT had failed to scan for HPV or check my markers for immunotherapy. I corrected that, and the results improved my staging from IV to II (survivability jumped 20~30%) while giving me an additional treatment option to consider.

Information is power!

I learned thousands of new medical terms and improved my understanding of all the tests, markers, and any treatment methods available anywhere in the world. Nothing left unconsidered ... nothing ever considered too granular or too deep ... No such thing as too much information.

I soaked it all up ... a crash course in my cancer.

The goal ... to be able to converse with any oncologist at "close to peer level" and dive into the weeds with them about their findings, recommended plans or any other considerations about my case while also being able to bring my own research or ideas to the table to share in meaningful discussion and exchange.

<u>Recommendation</u> ... By educating yourself in the jargon of the alternate universe of cancer you find yourself in, you're changing the value proposition of every interaction ... for yourself (better understanding = better decisions) and for the experts you will meet.

With serious effort you are also **taken** more seriously and therefore **treated** more seriously, speeding the uptake of learning immensely. You can vet your research with the oncologists you meet, and you can vet the oncologists with the knowledge you've gathered ... One of them will end up being the doctor who has your life in their hands, after all.

Another dynamic worth mentioning is you place yourself not as "a patient to be managed" but squarely in the middle of what is going on as the key member of the team. It eases the ability to somewhat steer the processes and outcomes to fit your goals.

Bring your "A game" ... everyone else will too.

⑤ <u>Self Advocacy</u>

I found amongst many other cancer patients a "passing of the cancer burden" to the doctor resigning to "just following orders". Some just give up on any care whatsoever.

In my mind, it is a surrender to fate, which clouds everything to follow and cannot bode well. Certainly the first steps of a cancer journey must not begin on fatalistic footing.

Having lead my own company all these years, of course I brought with me certain "habits". Doctors were merely advisors I may (or may not) ask to join **my team,** and my job was to know enough to get the best out of the team I would finally choose.

Seizing the leadership role not only correctly brings ultimate responsibility back on yourself but also empowers you with a sense of agency.

Even more audaciously I allowed myself to flirt with the idea ... "cancer is not happening to me ... rather ... "I am happening to cancer."

It's a kind of "radical optimism" ... and anyone would consider it delusional ... correctly so, really.

Yet from studies one can learn that one of the most powerful extenders of life is a positive mindset ... whether you have a reason to be or not ... it works.

Even then, I already set my mind on the goal of meeting the challenge head on and recovering stronger than ever.

Recommendation ... Take on full responsibility for "the project" and its successful outcome like your life depends on it ... because it does!

⑥ Decisiveness

Paths I considered included ... TORS (trans-oral robotic surgery), S.O.C. (standard of care ... ie. the prevailing medically approved therapy at time of diagnosis), naturopathy, Chinese medicine, immunotherapy, tomotherapy ... and, doing nothing.

I weighed each with odds of overall success and percentage of risk.

As a dispassionate calculation, the answer came to me quickly ... I would take a **hybrid** approach adopting principals of metabolic therapy together with S.O.C. to boost my odds.

S.O.C. in my case was concurrent chemo and radiation therapy.

Chemotherapy Plan = 3 x 100mg/m^2 cisplatin ... Day 1, Day 25, Day 50

Radiation Therapy Plan via linear accelerator delivering external beam radiation using IMRT and IGRT.

Treatment schedule = 7 weeks.

Dosing = 70gy left side, 50gy right side (generally speaking)

I used the same method to decide on the team of doctors and the equipment to be used.

Recommendation ... Research options with the lens of scientific studies that can inform best odds to achieve your goals. Also, consider your team's experience and interview them rigorously.

In my case, tomotherapy would have been the logical better choice but the available machines were only a few months in situ compared to the Linac that had been in operation for a few years. The newest, latest machine is not always "best" if the operators have only recently been trained on it.

In the moment of decision lock up your emotions and concentrate on the facts ... digging, referencing and counter checking from every angle.

⑦ Mitigation

Mountaineering is sport where success is not guaranteed, and the risk of death or injury is always present ... basically, it's the definition of "adventure". A thorough examination of success strategies and risk mitigation is a normal part of prep work.

Summiting is also only "halfway" ... Returning home alive and uninjured to loved ones is how success is measured.

Having chosen my treatment plan (i.e., "the mountain") I could put 100% concentration on mitigation and success strategies for before, during, and after my treatment.

Having already expressed 100% confidence in my oncology team on their ability to "kill the cancer" (i.e. "summiting"), I wanted to shift their attention to my bigger question ... "what's left of me after you're done?"

I had to refocus the team to Q.O.L. (quality of life) as the definition of success.

Through research and discussions with other HNSCC patients as well as my oncology team, I created a list of ALL the side effects of CRT (during and after) and came up with ways to reduce, eliminate, or recover better from each of them.

I didn't wait to see which problems came up during treatment, I prepared for all of them in advance. This level of preparation puts you mentally in a much stronger position as you're already ready to handle most anything. If an odd surprise occurs, rather than being bogged down on multiple fronts, there's bandwidth now in reserve to address it fully.

A couple highlights ...

Fasting ... I utilized Dr. Valter Longo's protocol during chemo sessions and sailed right through them without discomfort or the typical after damage aside from some tinnitus in the 6K MHz range.

Mometasone Furoate ... I learned about this from Scottish breast cancer patients and saved myself from the usual horrible skin damage and scarring that is typical with radiation therapy.

Exercise (5~10 kms run, calisthenics) ... I kept my daily routine throughout ... even the darkest weeks after CRT when symptoms peak. I've never met or heard of another patient who kept such a regimen.

There are many, many other mitigations I deployed.

Recommendation ... focus on the risks and failure points you might face and do all the things great and small you can to improve or eliminate them. The methods I found were not known to my oncology team. Since then, they've upgraded their patient care to include some of my methods.

⑧ Hallmarks & Benchmarks

Completing treatment, my attention turned to the aftermath part of the plan ... 3 key areas ...

1) Recovery / Q.O.L. ... Aside from handling acute pain for many weeks, post treatment can be described like suddenly aging 20 years in a few weeks.

A stoic might wryly quip, "it's very unpleasant".

One challenge was sarcopenia. I had to quickly increase protein and add many more weight bearing exercises. After exposure to toxic chemo and radiation, my body didn't respond as before. I had to rethink and retool **everything** just to stop a downward spiral and eke out gradual, wavering progress.

Something I've done over the years for mountaineering is what I call "adversity training" ... training under the worst conditions ... bad weather, odd times, starved, tired, sore, unwell, exhausted, etc. Desensitizing to hardship and harnessing willpower to carry on when it's miserable sharpens your mental game leaving an edge of grit that might save your life if plans go sideways on the mountain.

And so, grit was my very good companion during recovery ... I kept after it.

I thought to myself, what a great opportunity to rebuild everything from below zero ... best adversity training **ever**!

2 years later, suddenly one day, I felt like "myself" again ... a great umbrage had lifted. Although I'm managing chronic tinnitus, trismus, and xerostomia, I'm now as strong as ever thus keeping my promise to myself.

2) N.E.D. / R.F.S. (no evidence of disease / relapse free survival)

To address this I studied cancer from the "somatic mutation theory" to the "metabolic theory" and finally landed upon the "cell suppression theory" to guide my study of the hallmarks of cancer looking for strategies.

I settled upon a "functional medicine" approach of every possible lever for creating health and reducing barriers to health. There's a dozen or so things that I simplified into an easy to follow set of regular habits.

So far ... NED/RFS achieved.

3) Longevity ... exposure to high doses of ionizing radiation damages DNA and, as it endlessly replicates "bad dna copies," creates a downstream trophic cascade of an entire host of conditions/malaise that can be filed under the title "premature aging."

So I also researched the hallmarks of aging, and I leaned on epigenetics research to guide my path.

Broadly, a very good anti-cancer strategy is also a very good anti-aging strategy ... and vice versa. Still there are extra things one can do to steer gene expression in more youthful directions.

One area as a quick example ... diet.

I found so many foods with anti-cancer and anti-aging benefits that I started making up recipes from my continually growing list.

... and I've had some good results.

How do I know? Benchmarking.

Recently there's a fantastic amount of research in this area as well as many brilliant thought leaders running labs and publishing their trials.

By benchmarking your blood work, scans, and physical performance to a "younger standard," you can target and pursue the lifestyle behaviors that create a biological age below your chronological years.

When the hair I lost during treatment finally grew back, I was happy to see more color and less grey than before. NYU recently discovered this is because melanocyte stem cell motility is restored.

That bending epigenetics could give me this result at sites near the highest damage ... Well, it has encouraged me to continue pushing my exposome toward vibrant health.

Recommendation ... in the same way an accurate diagnosis helps steer correct treatment, understanding the hallmarks of cancer and benchmarks of longevity yields clear targets to build and manage long-term health.

⑨ <u>Plans</u> & <u>Projects</u> ...

During my recovery, I put time into new plans and projects. Besides being a handy distraction, I found this life affirmingly therapeutic.

Of particular interest has been anything involving creativity, new skills acquisition, travel, and helping others.

<u>Recommendation</u> ... if you've fallen off your horse, the best thing is to shake it off and get back on your horse.

⑩ <u>Humor</u> ...

When facing a dire situation, keeping a sense of humor about yourself is useful on so many levels. Far beyond the cathartic effects, the health benefits are also well documented.

While you're laughing your way to better health, you're also helping all those who care about you to destress a notch or two.

When asked how I'm doing, I like to say something like ... "oh, worst hangover EVER!" ... or ... "hey, I don't need a nightlight anymore since I glow in the dark now!" ... or ... "ha! such a great way to lose weight ... would you like an introduction?"

I also concocted a brief "story" to amuse my friends while recovering ...

You are welcomed at the front door of the CANCER CASINO CLUB with a personalized lifetime membership card ...

"There you go, sir! Please proceed to the bar for your "welcome drink."

Ahhhh, the welcome drink ... it's is always the same ole "Atomic Zombie Cocktail." They serve so many of them, they just keep it in a black bag behind the bar.

After sipping on that for a while, the bartender leans over with a wink to let you know the staff at the tanning salon await.

He assures you, "They have a wonderful, 7 week program of premium radiation all lined up guaranteed to make you glow!"

Once properly bronzed, you're allowed to wander around a bit getting to know the casino.

And so ... you study the tables, interview the dealers, calculate the odds, hone your acumen ... seizing advantage where you perceive it ... with guile and wile.

You stack the decks ... and hide the aces ... and load the dice ... you do whatever it takes to stay in the game ... hoping for a reprieve.

... however just like Hotel California ...

You can check-out any time you like ... but you can never leave!

<u>Recommendation</u> ... sure, a serious mind guiding serious efforts is absolutely key ... but always remember to pair that with a light heart.

Note from Ann: I was mildly jealous reading Greg's story. He was able to craft an "equals" relationship with his MDs. He was clear they worked for him. Maybe I just hit the wrong clinics in the U.S., but the oncologists I ran into had less than zero interest in viewing me as an equal. Nope. I was a statistic. Perhaps, I'd have fared far better in China.

Ann's Story, Part 1

The words, "You have cancer," are ominous. No one wants to hear them. In late February 2021, about three weeks after my second Covid shot, I started bleeding. Not a big deal, except I was twenty years and then some into menopause. A special note here is I do not blame the covid vaccine for anything. Its link with menstrual abnormalities has been well established, and it may well have saved my life by encouraging my cancer to declare itself sooner than it would have absent the vaccines.

I'd taken bio-identical hormone replacement for over twenty years, and immediately quit. It was hard. Every symptom I'd been suppressing hit me with all the panache of a runaway train.

Night sweats.

Hot flashes.

Anxiety.

I made myself an appointment with an OB-GYN. It took her two tries to manage an endometrial biopsy. Since this is a procedure they learn as residents, and this woman was maybe thirty years into her practice life, it made me wonder about her general level of competence.

After she failed the first time, she sent me off for a trans-vaginal ultrasound. My endometrium was thicker than the five-millimeter standard, so I made an appointment for her to try another biopsy. This time, I told her that when I'd had the same procedure years ago, I'd been pre-medicated with Misoprostol. She obligingly wrote me an Rx for it, and it made the procedure possible. Excruciating, but possible.

Two weeks after the second attempt, Dr. Couldn't-Be-Bothered called me, uttered the horrible words, "You have cancer," and then proceeded to tell me she was new and had no idea where to refer me.

Oh, and I didn't have just any uterine cancer. Nope, I had an aggressive variety: serous carcinoma.

When I asked her, the expert, what my next steps should be, she said I needed to find a gynecologic oncologist and schedule surgery. She wasn't about to provide any direction or help beyond that. She also didn't schedule a follow up visit. I never heard from her again, which seemed strange. Even a lowly psychologist like me calls to check on how patients who've been given a life-threatening diagnosis are doing.

To figure out what to do next, I pulled up the yellow pages online. There was one gyn onc office, a long-but-doable drive from me. Because they were marginally closer than anywhere else, I called and scheduled an appointment.

I didn't get the main MD, the one who was an icon (in theory) in his field and who'd been in practice forever. Nope, I got shunted to his brand-new practice associate who'd just completed her gyn onc fellowship the previous year.

How bad could it be? I asked myself. Turned out the bad part was worse than my wildest imaginings, but I'm getting ahead of my tale. I did check her out through the medical licensing board in states where she held licensure and didn't unearth anything alarming.

Waiting is one of the hardest parts of this whole gig. While I waited, I did all the online research I could and ginned up a question list. It's how I operate. The more information I have, the better armed I am to come up with decent decisions.

Meanwhile, my husband and children were worried but trying for stiff upper lips. Ditto for my friends. I have more medical knowledge than virtually all of them—except the doctors—so they've always looked to me for guidance.

In this instance, I wanted someone to take care of me. Like maybe the MDs...

Yeah, it was like waiting for Godot. No one to take care of me, certainly not the MDs, although my PCP has been a gem throughout this mess of a journey. He's steadfastly believed in my right to make decisions for my body.

Even if he disagreed with them.

It bears repeating. He told me over and over he would support me no matter which path I chose. He believed I should get the full court press of chemotherapy. When I didn't feel that way, he didn't abandon me.

Agency over one's body should be a slam dunk, but it's not. I was fired from an infusion center for asking too many questions and taking too many supplements. More on that experience when we get there.

I did circle the wagons. Got on a list to begin acupuncture. It took over three months to secure my first appointment, but it was well worth the wait. I still go weekly. I looked up a psychotherapist I'd spent many hours with and resurrected my relationship with him. I relied on a doctor of Chinese medicine in the Bay Area to alter my supplement regimen in light of my new diagnosis. And I breathed life into my badly neglected meditation practice.

I started a nightly gratitude journal and bought a rebounder. I spent time in my far infrared sauna.

As a sidebar, one of the questions you ask yourself is how in the hell did I get cancer to begin with? No one in my immediate family has ever had it. No one. I was the first.

I've been a lifelong athlete, always eaten well. I don't drink or use drugs. My weight is normal. I've never lived in a high pollution area. As it turns out, I don't have any of the genetic underpinnings that can make a person prone to cancer like BRCA or KRAS.

So how did this happen to me?

I was well over a year into my cancer journey before I found out. I blamed the bioidentical hormones I'd taken for twenty plus years from the gate, but it's worse than that. My bioidenticals were transdermal, which means I smeared cream on my skin. A mix of estrogen and progesterone in the evening and testosterone in the morning.

I probably would have been fine, except transdermal progesterone is pretty worthless. What I should have been taking to oppose the estrogenic tendency to build up the uterine lining (hyperplasia), was micronized progesterone, an oral tablet.

You would think the long-ago OB-GYN who started me on that regimen would have known better. Nope. Essentially, I took close-to-unopposed estrogen for better than twenty years. Not enough to make me bleed except for one episode a few years in, but enough to sow the seeds of eventual disease.

No wonder I ended up with cancer.

There is a take-home message here. You have to do your own research. Just because someone has MD after their name, does not by itself mean they know everything, or that they can be trusted to come up with what is best for you.

The doctor whose prescription probably gave me cancer was supposedly an expert in hormone replacement therapy. He had years to correct my prescription, but he never did.

In case it sounds like I'm blaming him, I'm not. If there is fault, it lies with me for not doing better research about something that was leaching into my body through my skin over the long haul.

Physicians have never been gods, but they used to do a better job navigating the challenging waters of what to prescribe. Today, Big Pharma is a major player in that decision-making process. They're all about profit—double digit or better these last two decades.

Quite an accomplishment, and awesome for their stockholders. But any profit-driven motives come with collateral damage. Let's take a look at a couple more survivor stories before we tackle the big business cancer treatment has turned into.

Peta's Story

In June 2015 I was diagnosed with ER positive breast cancer in my right breast. That diagnosis was changed after CT scans & 2 Full body MRI scans. On 30th August 2015, my full diagnosis became stage 4 metastatic breast cancer, with nodes in my lung & lesions on my bones....pelvis, back bone, legs & ankles.

I decided not to accept any treatment from them. As my diagnosis was terminal, they couldn't cure me but could give me some extra time. I had not seen an oncologist at this point & the breast surgeon had booked me in for surgery on Friday 25th September....I told them that I didn't want surgery, but would go home & think about it. I left them dismayed in the consultation room & a nurse asked me if I wanted to die as I was refusing surgery.....& so the bullying began. I walked out of the hospital feeling elated....as for once in my life I followed my intuition....which told me to get out of there....I didn't need any of their treatment..... In the car park the elation turned to

"Fuck.....what have I just done".....so I looked skyward & asked for a sign that I had done the right thing......I thought to myself what was the most unlikely thing to happen to me at the moment.... The answer came to mind as 2 tickets to watch England play in the imminent Rugby World Cup, hosted by England. (During my childhood & teenage years my Dad played rugby.....it's a very social game & a lot of friends & relations were involved in it.) So I set that in my mind....about a week later I was offered 2 Tickets for England v Australia.....3rd October 2015, for free...(worth a very large sum of money) So here was my sign....very direct & completely on point & so my bizarre beautiful journey began.

I contacted the hospital & spoke to the breast surgeon to say I would not be taking up their offer of a mastectomy. She was aghast....however I did agree to meet with an oncologist in October to discuss my diagnosis....so even with my diagnosis I had to wait nearly 4 months to see an oncologist!

On Oct 3rd 2015....I headed to Twickenham, London England, with my friend Teresa & my sister Sarah to meet up with Orli & go to the Rugby game......it was a fabulous day full of laughter & mischief.....unfortunately England lost heavily to Australia.....hey ho.... I was still alive & living life to the fullest..... That became my mantra.....to really live my life.....I learnt the true meaning & healing powers of the word NO. I was no longer going to say yes, when I really wanted to say no. No more people pleasing, I was learning to please me with gusto! For a number of years I had had ongoing problems with Candida & had learnt to heal using herbs & diet.....so I knew that I would have to completely change my diet & that this would be ongoing, & would change with my body's needs... I knew the power of meditation, self-talk, qi gong, yoga, being in nature & embracing joy. I also knew the healing powers of connection & group therapy....& so I embarked on a program to heal me. I had created over many years & traumas the imbalance in my body, so I believed I could create the conditions in my body that would reverse that imbalance. I read numerous books all of which seemed to "find me" at the right time that I needed their author's wisdom....I came to see them as sign posts I was heading in the right direction & also they rerouted me a couple of times.

I was feeling the fittest & the best I had felt in years when I was given my diagnosis....so I kept my diet & fitness levels up.....my bones felt better when I did heavy weights & I loved cardio..... Meanwhile I got to see an Oncologist....It didn't go well.....but on the other hand it went brilliantly....as she got my back up....poopooing everything I was doing & said "did I really think I could heal myself"....so I picked up the gauntlet she had thrown me, but at the same time I did agree to take Tamoxifen, I would keep inside with them to get my scans.....

I tried Tamoxifen & gave it 3 months & really didn't like the effect of it on me.....I had another 2 scans before I stopped taking it. I tried on numerous occasions to contact the Oncologist but couldn't get to speak to her....so just stopped taking it..... When I saw her for my scan results, she told me there was now a lesion on my liver.....& I asked her how sure she was about that.....she replied I am 90% sure. I always took a friend with me to every meeting with them.....it helps to get a full picture when your emotion is high if it's a bad result.....

I learnt the word scanxiety......so it was good to have another soul & a pair of ears! I also asked her if she had ever really read up about Tamoxifen, & how it changes the liver function.....she replied no. I told her I had stopped taking it & she was furious. Also my breast tumor had increased, which I wasn't surprised as I had lost my mum 3 months before the scan & that had brought a lot of stress & deep emotions to the surface.

I agreed to have another scan in November 2016. My results for the November scan kept being delayed....so I knew in a funny way it was good news...so I finally got the results 6 weeks after the scan.....I took my friend Caroline who had been with me for the last meeting with my Oncologist & very glad I did!

In the room were my Oncologist, the Breast Surgeon & a Macmillan Nurse.... Ah the good news said my Oncologist....the lesion on your liver has disappeared & we don't think the bone lesions are cancer! OK so Tamoxifen looks like it caused the blip on the liver.....& when I stopped taking Tamoxifen it went away.....No said the Oncologist. OK so my bone lesions, you don't think are cancer, so what are they? Reply from my oncologist was "We don't know.".... You don't know but you do know that it isn't cancer...why? Because they aren't behaving like cancer..... I then asked as the "host" do I behave like your normal cancer patient.... They all replied NO.... I replied then that maybe is your answer....

I asked if it was rheumatoid arthritis? No. Osteoporosis with spurs No.... She said the delay meeting with me had been getting consultations on the results..... So I was then being forced to have a mastectomy as my cancer wasn't terminal as they had 1st diagnosed it..... They also said it needed to be next week otherwise it may be too late. So I was being pressurized into saying yes as they were concerned that there would not be enough skin & tissue to close me up & I could bleed out,.... There is no way I could hide the laugh that was bubbling up inside me....so I laughed..... I said to my Oncologist..."You should know by now I don't do fear, I will go home & in a quiet space think about what you have offered & whether it is for me."

I never went back & I have not had a scan since 2016. I saw my Oncologist in the hospital corridor in August 2017. She did say I looked very well....& told me I should come to her & ask her for what she could give me.....I said I wouldn't as I had actually decided to move to Turkey. I completely had the right Oncologist for me & the right diagnosis or misdiagnosis...... Had I just been diagnosed with breast cancer....I may have gone the conventional route......so even my bone misdiagnosis (if it is a misdiagnosis) still don't know what they are today.....all helped in guiding me to where I am now.....sitting in the glorious sunshine, surrounded by 5 rescued street dogs in the beautiful ancient Aegean area of Turkey.....

There is more....I sold my home gave up my business & bought a Citroën C3 Pluriel & drove to Turkey from England.....I landed in France on Valentine's Day 2018......drove through France, Italy, & Greece into Turkey....& here I am 8 years after.... There is still a tumor in my breast & I still have lesions on my bones.....but since I haven't had a scan since 2016 I have no idea how they're doing......I continue to feel well and enjoy each day.

Debbie's Story

After several months of lower right quadrant pain, I went to my doctor. He ordered an abdominal CT scan and lab work.

Results showed what they said looked like a malignant 9.5cm mass in the right lower abdomen. Labs were just as bad. My CEA was 12 and I was anemic.

I instinctively knew to stop all sugar, white flour and processed foods. When I heard the term "stage 4" I knew it was life or death. So I quit my job to focus all my energy on fighting to live.

After a colonoscopy it was determined by my colorectal surgeon I should have surgery right away. Two weeks later they removed 3 ft of my colon, my cecum and my appendix. Malignancy was verified by the Pathologist.

Next stop was the Oncologist. He gave me 4 weeks to recover from surgery and then started me on IV chemotherapy. Folfox and Oxaliplatinum. Which made me very lethargic and nauseated. The weight fell off and I slept a lot. I lost 75 pounds in 8 weeks.

I prayed for direction, then books, literature and testimonies started falling into my path. Along with my prayer regimen I read insatiably. I also researched for a good Naturopathic practitioner in my area. I ended up at a naturopathic doctor in the town I live in. After reviewing my history she said, "You don't need me. You need to see my colleague, Dr Sean Devlin."

Immediately, I made an appointment with Dr Devlin. His office is a 4 hour round trip from my house. I would make the trip 3 days a week. He put me on a regimen of IV artesunate, high dose Vitamin C, and mistletoe. This regimen continued for several months concurrently with the treatment prescribed by my Oncologist.

Over the next 12 months the cancer spread to my liver and right lung. The Hepatic surgeon took out 3 sections of my liver and the Pulmonary surgeon took out the right upper lung. After 4 weeks of recovery from each surgery the Oncologist put me back on IV chemotherapy.

When on a break from conventional therapy my husband and I found an RV park 10 minutes from Dr Devlin's office. We scraped together enough funds to cover 7 weeks of intensive naturopathic treatments. My husband took me to Dr Devlin 5 days a week for 7 weeks. I would sit in the infusion center for 6-8 hours a day on IV's. We would play cards and listen to music to pass the time while the natural substances would drip drip drip into my veins.

Along with this natural medicine therapy I completely changed my diet and lifestyle. I became a vegetarian over night. I would walk 1-2 miles a day. I also practiced stress reduction and relaxation techniques using slow deep breathing.

Thankfully, Dr Devlin had read the same books as me on fighting cancer metabolically. He prescribed off label medications that Pub Med studies have shown kill cancer. At this point he had me taking Metformin, aspirin, atorvastatin and Loratadine every day along with many plant supplements which block cancer from entering cell pathways. I also continued the IV therapies he prescribed. I did all this along with conventional IV chemotherapy.

This all happened over the course of 2 years. Because insurance would not pay for the naturopathic treatments, we had to get a second mortgage on our home, do a Go Fund Me, take all our 401K and savings to pay for Dr Devlin's care. Again thankfully, my husband and children were very supportive. They said they would rather have me than the money. I'm very blessed to be loved so much.

During this time I came close to death on more than one occasion. Hospitalized at one point to receive 3 units of blood due to a critical hemoglobin value of 5.

At Christmas my blood pressure fell to 80/30. Again put in the hospital for supportive measures until my body could get strong enough to keep fighting. During this hospitalization my family called our pastor to pray over me. He prayed for healing and strength.

At 2 1/2 years into this journey I got a clear whole body PET scan and my CEA dropped to 2.0. At this point my husband asked the Oncologist what's next? Her response was, "I don't know. I never expected you to get to this point."

I'm now 4 years from the date of diagnosis and still cancer free. Dr Devlin (who is the only doctor I give credence to in cancer treatment) has given me the target of March 2025. This is my "cure" date. My goal is to stay NED until that date. Then we will celebrate!!!

Until then I continue the off label drugs Dr Devlin prescribed, high dose IV Vitamin C, my plant supplements, a vegetarian diet, daily exercise and stress management. I also take high doses of melatonin at bedtime and pray, pray, pray to stay healthy.

This is my story. I'm very aware many others have a similar story and didn't make it. I do not take survival lightly. I know because I lived God must have a plan for my life. My desire is to know that plan and live it out to His glory, so my life is not lived in vain.

Cancer is Big Business

Cancer is big business in America. How big, you might ask? To the tune of billions of dollars. Let's take a peek at a few statistics.

In a study from the University of North Carolina at Chapel Hill reproduced in the Journal of Oncology in 2017, researchers looked at the relationship between pharmaceutical company payments to oncologists and the likelihood of them prescribing a particular cancer-related drug. Here is an encapsulation of the results of that study:

"Receipt of general payments from pharmaceutical companies is associated with increased prescribing of those companies' drugs. An association between research payments and prescribing was less consistent. This study suggests that conflicts of interest with the pharmaceutical industry may influence oncologists in high-stakes treatment decisions for patients with cancer."

In plain English, that means Big Pharma pays for the privilege of making certain their drugs are up close and personal. At the forefront of prescribing MD's minds.

I want to highlight another Big Pharma practice. It's basically gaming the U.S. patent system to protect lucrative monopolies on blockbuster drugs. The process of patent extension strategy goes like this. A drug company has a multi-million-dollar successful drug that's toward the front end of its twenty-year patent. Meanwhile, research scientists in their lab come up with a better version. It could be safer with fewer side effects, or it might have a simpler route of administration. For example, subcutaneous injection rather than intravenous. Instead of hustling the better version to market, the drug company instructs its research division to sit on it so it won't be competition for the drug that's already out there until much closer to it being off patent.

This sketchy practice has a name: product hopping. Drug companies want to maintain their monopoly on a medication. Just before the patent runs out (and generics are allowed to copy the formulation), they switch patients to their brand new, recently patented version of a similar drug. Timing is everything.

Hard to believe, but this really happens. As of the current date (July 2023) Gilead Sciences is being sued for this practice by a large group of AIDS patients for withholding a safer version of an antiviral for ten years.

Merck is engaged in something similar with Keytruda, their very successful immunotherapy drug. They've developed a version that can be administered subcutaneously. It will extend the company's revenue stream for years after the original patent expires in 2028.

In the U.S. physicians are supposed to report payment of more than $10 from drug companies, but there is no prohibition against them taking kickbacks from Big Pharma. Except they don't call them kickbacks. Nope. It's a dirty word. Those payments are called "incentives."

Back in the days when I taught at a family medicine residency, we didn't have so much as a Kleenex box that didn't have some drug name on it. The pharm reps used to buy lunch for the entire residency every Wednesday in exchange for a quarter hour to pimp the latest and greatest wonder drug. The drug companies also sponsored movies, fancy meals, golf, and even entire vacations for physicians.

More of the same from one more doctor and another study:

"If there are physicians out there that deny that there is a relationship {between the money they receive from pharmaceutical companies and their prescribing practices, they are starting to look more and more like climate deniers in the face of the growing evidence," said Aaron Kesselheim, a professor of medicine at Harvard Medical School and an expert in pharmaceutical costs and regulation. "The association is consistent across the different types of payments. It's also consistent across numerous drug specialties and drug types, across multiple different fields of medicine. And for small and large payments. It's a remarkably durable effect. No specialty is immune from this phenomenon."

Both Big Pharma and MDs consider this "grease the palms" arrangement a win-win.

Too bad the losers are their patients. If an older drug, with a proven track record of non-toxicity, will do the trick, why subject patients to something newer that's many times more expensive?

Those new drugs sometimes don't make it past a couple of years on the market before they're either withdrawn or given black box warnings because they've killed too many people.

But MDs keep on prescribing them. The sad truth is many of them have closer relationships to pharm reps than they do to their patients.

Back to cancer.

According to Robert Nagourney, MD, founder of the Nagourney Cancer Institute, only one out of seven clinical trials actually shows that A is better than B in terms of treatment. Only one out of fourteen clinical trials improves survivability by more than 50 percent.

Even this is a deceptive statistic. If drug A provides progression free survival (PFS) of two weeks, and drug B provides three weeks, it meets Dr. Nagourney's criteria. The sad truth is hardly any of the new drugs increase PFS by more than a couple of months.

The "war on cancer" has been ongoing for well over half a century. It's only recently we've come up with new weapons in the arsenal that can actually work far better than chemotherapy for selected patients. A problem is drug companies do not want to give up their lucrative chemotherapy infusions.

Nope. Even when an immunotherapy has been proven to work better with far less toxicity, getting it through the FDA as an approved first-line treatment takes years. Meanwhile, everyone stuck with old-school chemo agents could be receiving second-rate medicine.

Second-rate medicine that is trashing their immune systems and wreaking other havoc in their bodies. Chemo doesn't touch cancer stem cells—it may actually strengthen them—and they are a primary source of metastases.

No one knows, absent genomic/molecular testing, what drug will actually attack a particular cancer. Genomic/molecular testing should happen first, before any treatment, not as an afterthought when treatment has failed.

No one seems to care. Or even appreciate it's a problem.

Let's fill in some figures for just how lucrative cancer treatment is.

The following is from an article by John Horgan in Scientific American, February 12, 2020.

Since Mr. Horgan covers all the bases, with his express permission, I'm going to excerpt large sections from that article. The title is "The Cancer Industry: Hype Versus Reality." It kind of says it all. Forgive me since it's long, but there are pearls scattered throughout. Those reading the paperback can pull up the original article online to follow hyperlinks of interest.

. . .

"First, some basic facts to convey the scale of the problem. Cancer is the second most lethal disease in the U.S., behind only heart disease. More than 1.7 million Americans were diagnosed with cancer in 2018, and more than 600,000 died. Over 15 million Americans cancer survivors are alive today. Almost four out of ten people will be diagnosed in their lifetime, according to the National Cancer Institute.

Cancer has spawned a huge industrial complex involving government agencies, pharmaceutical and biomedical firms, hospitals and clinics, universities, professional societies, nonprofit foundations and media. The costs of cancer care have surged 40 percent in the last decade, from $125 billion in 2010 to $175 billion in 2020 (projected).

Research funding has also surged. The budget of the National Cancer Institute, a federal agency founded in 1937, now totals over $7 billion/year. That is a fraction of the total spent on research by nonprofit foundations, private firms, and other government agencies. Total research spending since Richard Nixon declared a "war on cancer" in 1971 exceeds a quarter trillion dollars, according to a 2016 estimate.

Cancer-industry boosters claim that investments in research, testing, and treatment have led to "incredible progress" and millions of "cancer deaths averted," as the homepage of the American Cancer Society, a nonprofit that receives money from biomedical firms, puts it. A 2016 study found that cancer experts and the media often describe new treatments with terms such as "breakthrough," "game changer," "miracle," "cure," "home run," "revolutionary," "transformative," "life saver," "groundbreaking" and "marvelous."

There are more than 1,200 accredited cancer centers in the U.S. They spent $173 million on television and magazine ads directed at the public in 2014, according to a 2018 study, and 43 of the 48 top spenders "deceptively promot[ed] atypical patient experiences through the use of powerful testimonials." A 2014 study concluded that cancer centers "frequently promote cancer therapy with emotional appeals that evoke hope and fear while rarely providing accurate information about risks, benefits, costs, or insurance availability."

LITTLE NET PROGRESS AFTER 90 YEARS, BESIDES ANTI-SMOKING EFFORTS

What's the reality behind the hype? "No one is winning the war on cancer," Azra Raza, an oncologist at Columbia, asserts in her 2019 book *The First Cell: And the Costs of Pursuing Cancer to the Last*. "Claims of progress are mostly hype, the same rhetoric from the same self-important voices for the past half century." Trials have yielded improved treatments for childhood cancers and specific cancers of the blood, bone-marrow, and lymph systems, Raza notes. But these successes, which involve uncommon cancers, are exceptions among a "litany of failures."

The best way to measure progress against cancer is to look at mortality rates, the number of people who succumb to cancer per unit of population per year. The risk of cancer grows with age. (Although childhood cancer gets a lot of attention, Americans under 20 years old account for less than 0.3 percent of all U.S. cancer deaths.) Hence as the average life span of a population grows (because of advances against heart and respiratory disorders, infectious disease, and so on), so does the cancer mortality rate. To calculate mortality trends over time therefore, researchers adjust for the aging of the population.

With this adjustment—which, keep in mind, presents cancer medicine in a more favorable light—mortality rates have declined almost 30 percent since 1991. This trend, according to cancer-industry boosters, shows that investments in research, tests, and treatments have paid off. What boosters often fail to mention is that recent declines in cancer mortality follow at least 60 years of *increases*. The current age-adjusted mortality rate for all cancers in the U.S., 152.4 deaths per 100,000 people, is just under what it was in 1930, according to a recent analysis."

NEW TREATMENTS YIELD SMALL BENEFITS, BIG COSTS

"Research has linked cancer to many internal and external factors, notably oncogenes, hormones, viruses, carcinogens (such as those in cigarettes), and random cellular replication errors, or "bad luck." But with the notable exception of the smoking/cancer link, which led to effective anti-smoking measures, that knowledge has not translated into significantly improved preventive measures or treatments. Clinical cancer trials "have the highest failure rate compared with other therapeutic areas," according to a 2012 paper.

Pharmaceutical companies keep bringing new drugs to market. But one study found that 72 new anticancer drugs approved by the FDA between 2004 and 2014 prolonged survival for an average of 2.1 months. A 2017 report concluded that "most cancer drug approvals have not been shown to, or do not, improve clinically relevant end points," including survival and quality of life. The authors worried that "the FDA may be approving many costly, toxic drugs that do not improve overall survival."

I'm going to insert a comment here. For my type of cancer, there is convincing longitudinal research that proves radiation doesn't improve outcomes, yet radiation remains part of the standard of care for treatment of uterine cancer. My question is why? Radiation has its own set of problems and can cause other cancers years down the road.

Back to Mr. Horgan's well-researched article.

"Costs of cancer treatments have vastly outpaced inflation, and new drugs are estimated to cost on average more than $100,000/year. Patients end up bearing a significant proportion of costs. More than 40 percent of people diagnosed with cancer lose their life savings within 2 years, according to one estimate.

Immune therapies, which seek to stimulate immune responses to cancer, have generated enormous excitement. Two researchers won the 2018 Nobel Prize for work related to immune therapies, and a new book, *The Breakthrough:*

Immunotherapy and the Race to Cure Cancer, claims that they represent a "revolutionary discovery in our understanding of cancer and how to beat it."

According to a 2018 report in *Stat News*, drug firms aggressively market immune therapies, and patients are "pushing hard to try them, even when there is little to no evidence the drugs will work for their particular cancer." A 2017 analysis by oncologists Nathan Gay and Vinay Prasad estimated that fewer than 10 percent of cancer patients can benefit from immune therapies, and that is a "best-case scenario."

Immune therapies can trigger severe side effects, and they are also extremely expensive, costing hundreds of thousands of dollars a year. Oncologist, Siddhartha Mukherjee, author of *The Emperor of All Maladies*, a bestselling history of cancer, reported in the *New Yorker* last year that "Subsequent hospital stays and supportive care can drive the total costs to a million dollars or more. If widely prescribed, immune therapies "could bankrupt the American health-care system."

Mr. Horgan goes on to discuss how a lot of cancer screening yields false positive results, but the section of his report that circles back to the beginning of this chapter has to do with corruption.

CORRUPTION IN THE CANCER INDUSTRY

"The aggressive, can-do American approach to health care isn't working when it comes to medicine in general and cancer medicine in particular. The U.S. spends far more per capita on health care, including cancer care, than any other country, but higher expenditures have not led to longer lives. Quite the contrary. Europe, which spends much less on cancer care than the U.S., has lower cancer mortality rates, according to a 2015 study. So do countries such as Mexico, Italy and Brazil, according to Our World in Data."

Let me insert a comment here. Europe, Mexico, Brazil, etc. include non-toxic interventions like intravenous vitamin C and mistletoe to treat cancer. My opinion as to why we don't use them here is because Big Pharma can't profit off them. Okay, back to Mr. Horgan.

"The American approach fosters corruption. According to a 2019 essay in *Stat News* by oncologist Vinay Prasad, many cancer specialists accept payments from firms whose drugs they prescribe. This practice "leads us to celebrate marginal drugs as if they were game-changers," Prasad argues. "It leads experts to ignore or downplay flaws and deficits in cancer clinical trials. It keeps doctors silent about the crushing price of cancer medicines."

Last year *The New York Times* and *ProPublica* reported that top officials at Sloan Kettering Cancer Center "repeatedly violated policies on financial conflicts of interest, fostering a culture in which profits appeared to take precedence over research and patient care." Sloan Kettering's chief medical officer, Jose Baselga, "failed to disclose millions of dollars in payments from drug and health care companies in dozens of articles in medical journals." Baselga left Sloan Kettering to become head of cancer research at the drug firm AstraZeneca.

Note from Ann: Investigators must disclose conflicts of interest at the end of all published research articles. To conveniently leave something like that out is a serious ethical breach.

"The desire of oncologists to produce monetizable findings might also compromise the quality of their research. A 2012 examination of 53 "landmark" cancer studies found that only six could be reproduced. The so-called Reproducibility Project: Cancer Biology has examined 14 more recent highly cited studies, and has confirmed only five without qualification."

Hopefully, you're still reading. Horgan's paper is chockfull of useful information, particularly if you're following the hyperlinks. Synopsizing his article so far, despite billions spent, we're no further along in the "war on cancer" than we were back in 1970. In some ways, we're worse off, but you'd never know it to read the hype from Big Pharma.

One critical part of Horgan's paper details the billions spent on new drugs. Most are useless. A few extend PFS (progression free survival) by a couple of months. The cost to patients is high since side effect profiles are grim.

Against that backdrop, one would think oncologists would welcome all the help they could get from novel approaches like genomic testing, molecular testing, identifying mutations, and blocking metabolic pathways.

Again, nope.

The sad part of all this is patient care has taken a distant backseat. I experienced that firsthand as have countless other patients caught up in dealing with this disease.

First and foremost, cancer patients are terrified. No one wants to die before their time. So we get guilt-tripped and fear-tripped into treatments that destroy our immune systems, do nothing to address cancer stem cells (why cancer resurfaces), and create disabilities that will be with us for the rest of our lives.

Most of the traditional oncologists I came across didn't care about side effects. Or permanent problems. Their bully pulpit is that you finish treatment, no matter how sick it makes you, and no matter if their treatment does nothing to address your cancer.

More on that in subsequent chapters.

Let's return to my story in the next chapter.

Ann's Story, Part 2

I finally had my surgical consult with the junior doctor in a nearby city. To her credit, she answered my questions and sent me off for a CT. No one warns you, but the average CT packs about the same amount of radiation as 200 x-rays. Radiation can kill you. It can also cause you to develop new and different cancers years down the road, so you really want to limit your exposure.

The other trap with CTs is IV contrast. For a while there, they were scanning me at the drop of a hat. So much so, my kidney function went south. It took about eighteen months after I started refusing contrast for them to recover. What they fail to tell you is once you have had a no contrast CT, you have something for them to use to compare the next one to. I'm not a total rebel, though. I do drink the barium.

The original scan showed minimal uterine involvement and cysts on both ovaries.

Because I thought I should, I scheduled a second opinion in Sacramento. Back during my residency days, I worked for Sutter Health, so I picked them as a known quantity.

And met another fresh out of fellowship MD.

A point of clarification here. To become a gynecologic oncologist takes a long time. There are the four years of med school, four more years of an OB-GYN residency, and a two-year fellowship on top of that.

The MD in Sacramento was young and earnest. When she got around to belaboring what would happen five years out if I had a recurrence, I kind of stopped listening. Someone should have told her that people's ability to absorb bad news is limited.

Mostly because of logistics, I went with the other group. I've chided myself time and again for that decision, but you don't get do-overs on this particular journey.

Surgery day was May 7, 2021. This is a tough surgery, despite being robotic. Still, no hospital stay. They booted me out of there about three in the afternoon, and hubby and I returned to a hotel. The next day, we drove home.

I was depleted, miserable, and in pain.

But I did the best I could to be up and moving believing it would speed my recovery.

Meanwhile, I'd consulted with a doctor of Chinese medicine I've known for years right after my diagnosis. He beefed up my supplement regimen, and I was swallowing bunches of pills to help regain my health. Both biopsies and surgeries stir up cancer cells. One of my supplements, modified citrus pectin, specifically bonds to cancer cells and moves them out of the body. Dr. Eliaz has conducted significant research on his Pectasol-C product.

I've always been ridiculously healthy. My only previous surgeries were a tonsillectomy when I was seven and a broken fibula back in 1994. Moldering around feeling like crap is tough.

It tried my patience.

Our daughter came and helped for the first week. As always, she was a godsend.

Meanwhile, no one called me with the pathology results. A week passed, then ten days. My PCP went to work through back-office channels at the hospital where I'd had surgery, and he got hold of the report the surgeon should have called me with. Turns out it had been available for several days. When I asked her why she hadn't called me, she seemed surprised the report had shown up. Interesting because it would have been sent to her first.

Overall, the report was promising. No spread to my lymph system or much of anywhere else beyond my endometrium (minimal) and both ovaries.

Despite everything, I didn't seem to be recovering like I thought I should. I had flank pain, and my energy wasn't great. You'll remember the OB-GYN who steadfastly said she had no idea where to refer me or how to help.

Of course, you remember her.

I decided it would be in my best interest to establish care with a different OB-GYN. Just in case. No way was I returning to the first one. An MD in a nearby town came highly recommended, so I called and made an appointment.

It was one of the best things I could have done. She was a gem. Compassionate and a good listener. Much like my PCP, she's been a staunch advocate, someone I can trust.

Four-and-a-half weeks after my surgery, urine started pouring out of me. I had no idea why, but I couldn't stop it. My PCP suggested many things, none of which worked. I bought pads and diapers and a waterproof mattress pad. Before it showed up, I was sleeping on towels with garbage bags under them.

I made several trips to the ER and had a bunch more CT scans. The upshot of all those scans and contrast is my kidneys went south. They're fine now, but they only recovered because I started refusing IV contrast and more scans. One of my labs, BUN, will probably never be normal again, but the rest of them are.

I'm getting off track here.

During one of many ER visits, three MDs poured over the CT trying to figure out why urine was gushing out of me. They called the surgeon. I will never be certain, but I'm pretty sure she knew exactly what she'd done.

Did she tell anyone? Oh hell, no. If she'd said something, I'd have known what was wrong. So would the good doctors who were trying to help me.

Likewise, she never apologized to me or even acknowledged she'd done anything wrong. A simple apology would have gone a long way. We're all human. We make mistakes, but when we don't own them, they develop a life of their own.

I did make a trip up to her clinic where she examined me and pronounced I had a fistula. It's a new channel in the body, one that shouldn't be there. In my case, it was between my ureter and my vagina.

The surgeon never took responsibility, never apologized. Yeah, harping on that. Sorry.

What she'd probably done was get the heat tip of one of the robotic arms too close to my right ureter and fried it. Perhaps I've missed the proper nomenclature, but the DaVinci Robot seals incisions with sutures or with heat. It was the part of the robot that produced heat that I believe created my issue. I've had other MDs tell me one of the big downsides of robotic surgery is limitations to the visual field. I assume she couldn't see what she was doing.

I can be naïve, but it never occurred to me until her practice partner said, "Dr. X feels terrible about this," that I'd actually been the recipient of a major surgical fuckup.

Damn near everyone told me to sue.

I resisted.

Focusing on health and healing is incompatible with the anger needed to fuel a lawsuit, so I let it go. Perhaps it was a mistake because I found out through the grapevine she screwed up again.

Hopefully, this patient was able to have the damage repaired.

There could be more surgical mishaps, ones I don't know about. I've done a lot of soul searching about whether remaining silent was the proper path. Maybe if I'd spoken up, I could have saved the above-mentioned patient—and perhaps others—from a great deal of grief.

There are a lot of less-than-stellar surgeons out there. I'm sorry one crossed my path, but on the plus side, she did get all the cancer. Very little in this world is black and white.

The MD who never apologized told me I had to have the fistula repaired. She said they could thread a stent from my kidney to my bladder. Yeah. That didn't work. I ended up with a nephrostomy tube, which is a spike in my kidney that drained urine through a tube into a bag strapped to my leg.

That little uber fun procedure took two days at the hospital where I'd had surgery because the right hand didn't know what the left hand was doing. "My" doctor told me I'd only be there a few hours.

I was there so long, my ride had to leave. One of my family had to make a long car trip to drive me home. Four days later, black blood started pouring out of me. I was certain I was dying from complications from the nephrostomy tube.

Back to the ER I went at seven in the morning. Hell of a way to spend my anniversary.

The ER docs in Mammoth Lakes are heroes. Warm, compassionate, competent. They loaded me into an airplane.

I was airlifted to a nearby city, this time to a different hospital because I said I wouldn't return to the surgical hospital if it was the last one in the world.

After one more failed attempt to thread a stent from kidney to bladder and another nephrostomy tube, I ended up in yet one more robotic surgery six weeks after the first one to reimplant my right ureter. This surgery was much longer than the hysterectomy, so my anesthesia burden was much greater.

As a psychologist, I've certainly heard about mental aberrations because of anesthesia. Now I've experienced them. I was so anxious once consciousness returned, I would have curled into a ball and howled were I not hooked up to so many tubes.

I came out of that surgery with a Foley catheter and a stent from my right kidney to my bladder.

The Foley, which I wouldn't wish on my worst enemy, was there for three weeks. It gave me a chronic urinary tract infection that took two months to clear. I cycled through so many antibiotics, there probably wasn't a microbe left anywhere in my body.

Luckily, the OB-GYN I'd had the forethought to establish care with removed the Foley, so she spared me a trip to the nearby city. I'm not sure I could have managed a lengthy car trip with it in place. The stent stayed in my body for five weeks. It created flank and lower back pain but was much more tolerable than the Folsy.

Meanwhile, my left-a-lot-to-be-desired surgeon and her practice partner, Dr. Icon, were pushing chemo. Protocol says you're supposed to start it six weeks after the original surgery.

By now, I was pushing back hard. I told them no chemotherapy until I'd recovered from not one, but two, major surgeries.

The other little ripple, that wasn't so little after all, was what I call, "will the real surgeon please stand up."

After my botched hysterectomy, it won't surprise anyone that I requested Dr. Icon perform the second surgery and remove the stent. His office was really insistent regarding the junior associate performing stent removal. While on a phone call with her, I said I would far prefer having Dr. Icon do the stent removal since he was the one who'd done my second (successful) surgery reimplanting my right ureter.

I had extracted a promise from him prior to surgery that he would do it, and I had no reason to believe he hadn't.

During that phone call, the junior doctor proudly informed me my second surgery had been "hers" too. I was stunned. And furious. Dr. Icon had promised and then welched while I was unconscious and had no way to fight back.

It's a whole lot like being raped after someone poured Rohypnol into your drink.

For what it's worth, five minutes later, I fielded a second phone call from Dr. Icon to reassure me they'd done surgery number two "together."

Yeah, sure they did. I'd love to have been a fly on the wall to hear *that* conversation. The one that ensured after she admitted she'd spilled the beans.

I was forced to return to their office for stent removal. Dr. Icon didn't give me any flak and took it out. Good thing since no other office would touch their screw up. I know because I tried to talk a couple of urology groups into removing it.

After that, I moved on to a new gyn onc at Stanford. I found her approachable in that she at least listened to me. She, too, pushed chemo.

I kept on saying no. Once I felt a bit better, I went backpacking. Healing has mental as well as physical components. I was doing everything I could to reestablish "normal."

At the time, reclaiming my life felt far more important than subjecting myself to chemotherapy infusions.

Stay tuned for my next steps, but first I'm going to introduce you to another survivor.

Maria Wessling Bachteal's Story

I met Maria through Abbey Mitchell's Healing Cancer Study Support Group on Facebook. She is a functional nutritionist and the founder of Healing Nutrition of Sonoma. She has been in remission with no evidence of disease from Stage 4 HER2+ breast cancer since 2015, using an integrative approach that includes the best of conventional oncology and complementary therapies. In her consulting practice, Maria provides coaching on nutrition and lifestyle changes to women who are in remission from breast cancer, with a goal of regaining their health after treatment and reducing risk of recurrence. Maria also leads a Facebook group specifically for integrative approaches to HER2+ breast cancer as well as co-leading the Breast Cancer Pathways Group, which shares research on using off-label drugs and natural substances to block pathways important for the growth of breast cancer cells. As part of this effort, Maria and Abbey co-created a tool called the Breast Cancer Pathways worksheet that summarizes and categorizes research citations they have collected.

. . .

I live in Northern California about an hour and a half north of San Francisco on a beautiful property with views of vineyards, redwood trees, and mountains. I realize I'm incredibly fortunate and practice gratitude as part of my healing. I'm married with two adult children.

A scientist and editor by training, I spent many years working in publications for an environmental research organization. I've been interested in nutrition ever since experimenting with alternative diets in the 90s. Discovering that a gluten-free diet cleared up my lifelong digestive problems put me on my path to wellness. But not before encountering a few bumps in the road.

I went back to school and studied nutrition in 2011 right before and during my original breast cancer diagnosis. Several years passed before I was well enough to complete my studies and start a consulting practice.

In 2011 I was originally diagnosed Stage 2 Triple Positive breast cancer, nodes clear. Luckily for me I have great insurance and doctors who favor scans so I got a PET/CT after my surgery. Lo and behold I had a life-threatening additional primary tumor (ependymoma) in my spine C3-6. Instead of moving on to chemo for the breast cancer I endured a lengthy spinal surgery and a three week inpatient hospital stay that left me with significant numbness and loss of function in my hands and feet. But I survived and wasn't paralyzed, which had been a possible outcome.

During the months that followed I got three separate opinions on treating my breast cancer from oncologists. Remember, I had no evidence of disease after surgery and imaging. This was just "adjuvant" therapy. Despite the fact that I had newly growing nerves, no one seemed concerned about the risks of chemotherapy. I was particularly concerned about Carboplatin. My gut told me no but I wanted the targeted drug Herceptin but there seemed to be no way to get it without the standard Taxotere and Carboplatin chemotherapy. (Back then, it wasn't possible to get the current treatment of just a Taxane drug and Herceptin, or even just targeted therapy alone that's starting to gain acceptance.)

The port insertion prior to chemo was horrible and painful, so my first dose was delayed. When I finally got my first dose of chemo the side effects hit on Day 3—and they were worse than I could have imagined. Pain and electric shocks throughout my body had me writhing on a fetal position. After that I was "allowed" to stop the chemo but continue Herceptin. I also took an aromatase inhibitor every other day instead of daily, and augmented with natural estrogen modulators, as advised by an integrative oncologist.

The next three years were filled with visits to one specialist after the next, one drug after the next, trying to get relief from the pain. I even tried some very out of the box treatments, spending thousands of dollars. I developed extreme tingling in my left hand that seemed to be related to scar tissue from the port or delayed effects from the damage to my CNS from chemo. I was angry and in pain. It was a dark time.

Then in 2014 my markers started to rise and a PET/CT showed the cancer had spread to my liver and spine. Biopsies showed the cancer was no longer driven by estrogen, just HER2+. I was devastated but determined to beat this thing without more nerve damage. This time I employed the brightest consultants I could find and researched out-of-the box treatments. I had tumor sensitivity testing by Dr Larry Weisenthal and the Greek RGCC. The results validated each other. And guess what? Carboplatin showed 0% effectiveness in killing the cancer cells and Taxotere 25%. If I had agreed to standard of care again it would not have worked. I instead traveled to Reno, NV to Dr. James Forsythe, a board certified oncologist who did low-dose insulin-potentiated chemotherapy ("IPT"). After three rounds of IV drugs, other IV therapies, and two months of a lowered dose of oral chemotherapy, I had clean scans and my tumor markers were nearly normal. I also began targeted therapy for HER2+ breast cancer with my oncologist.

At that time, full response to treatment and remission from Stage 4 breast cancer was rare in conventional oncology.

Since 2019, I've been an active participant in several integrative cancer Facebook groups and started my own group for HER2+ breast cancer. As part of these efforts, I joined with fellow thriver Abbey Mitchell to create an interactive spreadsheet that summarizes the research we've found on off-label drugs and natural substances that block pathways that drive breast cancer. We offer this spreadsheet freely to our community.

Combining the recommendations of integrative cancer practitioners and doing my own my research on the cancer pathways important for HER2+ breast cancer, I put together a comprehensive protocol to support my continued remission.

I firmly believe if I had just followed the advice of my oncologist without seeking out other experts and taking an active role in my healing, I likely would have had another recurrence by now. I have maintained remission for 8 years as of 2023.

As a functional nutritionist by profession, I know that diet and lifestyle are powerful tools. I choose to combine the best of allopathic and evidence

-based herbal medicine and nutrition in my personal protocol. Lots of lifestyle changes too. Daily meditation, gratitude, and physical exercise are my "nonnegotiables."

My nutrition consulting practice focuses on functional nutrition, which gets to the root cause of chronic disease and helps people use food, nutritional supplements, and lifestyle changes to live better lives. I mainly work with breast cancer survivors who want to reduce their risk of recurrence. This work brings me great joy and purpose. Although I still carry the scars of a difficult journey and live with pain, I'm healthier and happier than I was before I heard the words "you have cancer."

Ann's Story, Part 3

I continued to be ambivalent about chemotherapy. By now, over three months had passed since my hysterectomy. My body was feeling strong again. My attitude was positive.

I had a couple of Zoom visits with the Stanford MD. And I examined the logistics of receiving chemotherapy from them. Stanford is about a seven-hour drive for me in the summer when the Sierra passes are open, and a ten-hour drive in winter.

Like many institutions, Stanford has rules. One is they don't farm out chemotherapy to other clinics. At least in theory, my little local hospital provides chemotherapy infusions.

More on that later.

As a compromise, I established care with yet one more MD, this one at an infusion center considerably closer to me than Stanford. She seemed nice enough at first. I scheduled my initial infusion in the middle of September with full transparency about my supplements and the other things I was doing to support my health.

If I were an MD, I would want to know what my patients were taking just in case something might be contraindicated with the array of drugs supporting chemotherapy.

I discovered later this was far from true. Cancer patients wiser than me counseled me to keep my mouth shut about anything "extra" I was doing to support my health.

My plan was to transfer the infusion aspect of my treatment to Mammoth Hospital once I'd had the requisite initial infusion and hadn't dropped dead from side effects.

Meanwhile, I researched cold-capping to try to retain my hair. I also purchased ice mitts and ice booties to hopefully avoid neuropathy, a known complication from chemotherapy. As a writer, I really need my fingers to function properly. Neuropathy in one's feet is truly miserable. I ramped up my nightly melatonin to 120 milligrams to hopefully circumvent the brain fog that often accompanies chemotherapy.

My initial infusion was on 9/17, over four months after my hysterectomy. The first two days post infusion weren't bad, but after that, things went downhill fast. I couldn't tolerate the steroid (Decadron) they wanted me to take. It made me feel like I wanted to rip the skin off my body. I even did a fast-mimicking diet (Valter Longo) beginning the day prior to chemo to mitigate side effects. Unfortunately, it didn't work for me.

I had the prescience to refuse the colony-forming factor, Neulasta, they tried to shove down my throat in a time-release injection. My reasoning was I wanted to sort out chemo side effects from everything else. It made sense to me to wait and see if my white cells took a nosedive. Turns out they didn't, so Neulasta, which comes with a boatload of difficult side effects including severe bone pain, wasn't needed in my case.

I'd purchased a veritable cancer library in the months since my diagnosis. Titles can be found in the resources section at the back of this book. Between them and PubMed, a free medical database maintained by the National Institute of Health, I discovered there were many possible infusion schedules beyond the one the MDs were trying to force me to adhere to.

At my next appointment with the infusion center oncologist, I showed up with my question list and a lot of ideas. That was the appointment where I drove three hours to see her, waited half an hour in her waiting room, and she dismissed me after less than five minutes.

Dismissal consisted of her standing and ushering me out of her office while I was still talking. Her final comment was she'd only agreed to see me as a favor to Dr. Icon. Really? Dr. Icon hadn't referred me to her. The Stanford MD had. That kind of says it all. She cared so little about me as a human being, she didn't even bother to get her facts straight.

I was in tears, but not until I got outside to my car.

Illegitimi non carborundum sort of means, "Don't let the bastards grind you down." I refused to let that MD know how badly she'd rattled me.

Before I knew how I'd react to chemotherapy, I'd connected with the local infusion nurse to ensure I could receive treatment five minutes from home rather than several hours.

That was a joke. She steadfastly said she'd never received orders from the infusion center despite me actually being in a room with the physicians's assistant while she faxed them. This was perhaps the sixth attempt on the part of the infusion center to send orders. They all fell into a black hole. The infusion center even called along the way to make certain they were faxing to the correct number.

In so many ways, my treatment was a total shitshow.

In others, I choose to believe someone was watching out for me. You'll find out why presently.

I got hold of the Stanford MD after the infusion center MD dismissed me and discussed alternative infusion schedules. The Stanford MD was fine with a lower albeit more frequent dose schedule and told me she'd confer with the infusion center MD.

Weeks passed. The local nurse totally blew me off. Didn't even return my phone calls. As a last-ditch effort, I messaged the MD she reports to and mentioned I'd love to have chemo locally. During one of my many, many trips to the ER between my two surgeries, he'd made a point of offering that service.

The nurse did finally call me then. She was vague and evasive but did admit she had the orders. Then she said, "We're such a small center. If we mix up an infusion for you, and you don't show up, it will cost us a lot." Seemed like a weird thing for her to say since they'd never even offered me an appointment for me to not be there for. Plus, I've never missed an appointment at my local hospital, so why she would highlight it as a potential problem made no sense.

Except to vindicate her actions.

Anyway, it didn't matter since she promised to get back to me and never did. Again. Somehow, it didn't surprise me. In truth, I wouldn't have trusted her to set up or monitor an infusion for me. Not after what had happened.

I attempted to move on to the hospital in Bishop. They were very nice—and they had no problem securing orders—but said I had to have a port, something I really didn't want.

I finally had infusion number two in November. It was full dose Carboplatin and a much-reduced dose of Taxol. And it was far more tolerable.

Remember, I live several hours from the infusion center. Double that round trip.

I couldn't make the next week's appointment, so I called and cancelled in plenty of time for them to fill my slot. My intention was to show up the following week.

Intentions aren't worth much, apparently.

I went into the patient portal for something or other only to discover I'd been wiped off the face of the earth. That clinic didn't have the simple decency to speak with me. Nope. They just X-ed me off their patient roster.

When I called to dig a little deeper, I only got to talk with someone because I was insistent. What she said was the MD wasn't comfortable providing "subpar" treatment.

Insert a major eye roll here. That particular MD had been trying to get rid of me ever since I questioned the standard of care dosing schedule.

If it were her body, she'd damn well have asked questions.

In her world, no treatment was better than me missing the occasional week.

I was devastated. Certain they'd signed my death warrant.

Let me add something here. Ditching patients is ethically sketchy, particularly when said patient's only "sin" was asking questions. I was always polite. I didn't roll into their lobby pitching fits. I didn't raise my voice. I didn't threaten anyone with firearms. Those are the usual reasons patients are rejected.

When you cut to the chase, she dumped me because she didn't like me. That's antithetical to the Hippocratic Oath. She doesn't get the luxury of picking and choosing her patients. That was the one point in my cancer journey when I actually considered legal action. I'm certain she didn't run ditching me past the phalanx of attorneys employed by her medical center. Had she done so, they'd have told her she lacked grounds to terminate me as a patient.

If they terminated every patient who wasn't totally compliant, they'd go broke.

Still, I didn't want to be drawn into negativity. Listening to her lie to cover her actions would have engendered stress I didn't need. In the end, I let it go. I'm not sorry. Given another chance, I'd do the same.

If felt like the entire world was working against me having chemotherapy. From the local nurse who lost, misplaced, or never received orders, to the Bishop hospital requiring a port, to the infusion center MD firing me.

In case I'm sounding kind of victim-like, let me correct that impression. I can be outspoken. I'm old and have opinions. It's tough to divert me, particularly when my life is on the line. Because relationships are always two-way streets, I'm certain my ambivalence bled through and was why I received the reactions I did from various doctors and institutions.

I get it about rules. No particular reason for anyone to bend theirs on my behalf. The only part of the shitshow that I didn't play into directly was the nurse's difficulty around receiving orders. The infusion center sent them multiple times. I can see one fax being lost or misplaced, but multiple ones?

Turns out the progression of events was an incredible gift, but it didn't seem like it at the time.

That night was the one and only time when I pulled out my gratitude journal, the one I wrote in every evening, said, "Piss on it," and stuffed it back into its drawer.

Let's look at another couple of survivor stories, shall we?

Mine has developed a few darker edges.

Angela's Story

My cancer story has been going on for longer than I care to think about. I was two years or so into my marriage when my father died. It was a protracted and thoroughly unpleasant experience for him as he spent six weeks in intensive care on a ventilator, unable to speak to his loved ones and getting ever weaker and less able to breathe. I distinctly remember feeling utterly powerless to do anything about his suffering and that feeling of helplessness shook me to the core.

Within a couple of years, at the age of 46, I was diagnosed with triple negative cancer in my left breast and in early 2007 had a mastectomy. I found the loss of my pretty little boob quite traumatic, and I remember crying as they wheeled me towards the operating theatre. I also remember mouthing 'it's the left one' and pointing at it to the staff as they put me to sleep. I didn't want them removing the wrong one! The experience was profoundly traumatic; like everyone else, I didn't think cancer would happen to me!

There followed a very difficult few weeks as my oncologist insisted I should have 5FU chemotherapy. After much soul searching I declined and she completely washed her hands of me, promising me I would die. I have never felt so alone on my journey through life. Although I am in the extremely lucky position of having a very supportive and loving husband, any decisions were and are mine and mine alone. This felt impossibly difficult at first. I was afraid and often panicky but over the years it has become easier to the extent that I wouldn't now have it any other way.

I did everything I could think of to rebuild my health. I had always thought of myself as healthy, making careful food choices and enjoying plenty of fresh air and exercise. As we were living in France at the time, I was probably enjoying a little too much red wine but I have never smoked and certainly had no other comorbidities. My weight was always at the low end of the healthy range and my energy was generally good. I tried going vegan, eating only raw food and various other restrictive diets but found that any restrictions made me instantly start losing weight which I really didn't want to do. Eventually I settled on the '80/20' diet, though it's actually more like '95/5'. I eat 95% good quality Mediterranean diet, including plenty of lentils and pulses and allow myself a treat when it seems appropriate. After all, I am surviving and thriving, not just getting by. So if a delicious dessert has been lovingly prepared by a friend, for example, I will enjoy it without a trace of guilt. A couple of glasses of red wine a week are good for me in my world and I seldom drink more.

I remained clear of cancer for 5 years until 2012 and was feeling celebratory, as if that milestone meant I was free of it. Then, following a frightening and traumatic personal financial crisis, I felt a lump in my other breast. This turned out to be an entirely different cancer rather than a recurrence. It was ER+ HER2-. Also it was lobular rather than ductal. I had surgery to remove the lump but unfortunately the margins were not clear so I had another operation, this time a second mastectomy. I had been flat on the left side for 5 years following my first mastectomy and found it difficult to deal with, so I went for a reconstruction on both sides. I had expanders put in and gradually over a period of several months they were blown up like bicycle tires. This was not a pleasant experience and was excruciatingly painful for a few hours after each increase. Eventually I had another operation to put in the final implants. This has been a good decision for me so far. They have given me no problems at all and I find it infinitely easier to dress how I want to. At least with my clothes on, I feel completely 'normal'! I was told that this particular cancer had a low Ki67 and therefore was unlikely to cause further problems. So I sighed a huge sigh of relief and got on with my life.

At the end of 2015 my mother was taken ill and was rushed to hospital. There followed the worst months of my life as it turned out that, unbeknownst to me, two other family members had been systematically asset-stripping my poor mum. She had been frantic with worry. The payments for her house, which she had sold to one of these two via a solicitor, were not being made. The other one had taken her bank details and set up online banking on her behalf (without her knowledge or permission) and was helping himself to her meagre life savings. She had been tricked into losing half her small pension each month to pay off a car loan when she thought she was simply acting as guarantor. I could write a book about the series of unfolding horrors that became apparent as my trusting, honest mum lay dying in hospital. She had chosen not to tell me anything about what was going on for several reasons; she felt foolish and upset about it, she was still hoping against hope that these two would sort everything out and pay her back, and she didn't want to create discord in the family. She was living with her sister, my aunt, up until going into hospital and even her own sister had no idea what was going on. She definitely lost all will to live and after three months in hospital, they finally decided she wasn't going to recover and removed her ventilator. It took her all day to die, and it was profoundly distressing for her and for me.

It is often said that breast cancer may follow a trauma in life and so it was with me, yet again. Within two years, I was diagnosed with stage 4 breast cancer. The second cancer (ER+) had spread to my liver, mesentery, skin and many bones. I was given to believe that I was dying. I was utterly shocked and spent the next three months or so in a terrible state of fear. I had seen people die of cancer, and the thought of following them was terrifying. I had also witnessed both parents suffer and die slowly in hospital. I did not want that fate for me. Besides, how would my husband manage without me? I knew for a fact he didn't want to be left alone and probably wouldn't cope well. Not to mention my beloved cat!

Then I read Jane McLelland's book 'How to Starve Cancer' and began to realise that a different fate may be possible. If she could do it, why couldn't I? I soon realised though that a lot had changed in the 15 years since Jane's recovery, and it wasn't going to be easy to source all the off-label drugs that she had managed to get hold of. I kept searching and found Joe Tippens' story. I began taking fenbendazole in addition to Letrozole. At the time I was also on Ibrance and Xgeva. Within a year all my cancer had disappeared (I make no claims for the fenbendazole here, I'm simply relating what happened to me.

Would Letrozole alone have achieved this for me? There is no way to know). That was 2018 and although I have had several scans since, none has shown any cancer. Ibrance was problematic for me, as I believe it often is for slim women. My white blood cells were always too low and my oncologists, in my view, were far too slow to reduce the dose, despite my frequent requests. Eventually, they decided it was doing as much harm as good and I came off it, with some relief. I ditched the Xgeva after a year as well because, after much research, I became convinced that while it was keeping my bones denser, it was likely also making them more brittle. I just was not comfortable taking this stuff long term. (Of course this is not advice to anyone else, simply my decisions).

So my only conventional medication these days is Letrozole. I have been taking it for several years now and have sometimes taken a break from it. I am currently taking a half dose. I don't feel ready to come off it completely and I am lucky in that I don't have too much in the way of side effects from it (although my tendons and ligaments are sometimes tight and sore).

I discovered the excellent work of Abbey Mitchell and Maria Wessling Bachteal about four years ago and have never looked back. They have put enormous effort into collating information about natural alternatives to some of the drugs that Jane McLelland has used to such good effect. They look at blocking various 'pathways' through which cancer develops and feeds itself, whilst also attempting to prevent resistance to aromatase inhibitors and other 'standard of care' drugs. I have spent a considerable sum of money on various supplements over the years and I am sure they have helped me maintain excellent health and energy. At the moment I am taking a break from many of them but am still taking high dose melatonin, CBD oil, a baby aspirin, black seed oil and omega 3 fish oil in addition to my half dose of Letrozole. My oncologist is completely disinterested in anything other than standard of care so this road is mine and mine alone. I am happy with that.

There is much more to this journey than medication and supplements, however. It took my third bout of cancer to realise this. Shortly after diagnosis I was staying with a friend and she asked if I wanted to accompany her to a Buddhist meditation that she went to each week. I went along and to my immense surprise, came out feeling so much better than when I went in. I had not realised how much tension I was holding in my body. Within a few minutes of being talked through a meditation, I felt more relaxed than I could remember. I researched this and realised that my rather tense, nervous personality meant that I was spending too much time stimulating the sympathetic nervous system ('fight or flight') so that the parasympathetic nervous system ('rest and repair') just wasn't getting a look in. I see now that the combination of my personality and various horrendous adverse life events had brought about a catastrophic health crisis. I literally had to change or die.

I had always tended to consider others before myself, to see others as more important than me. I had always felt inadequate on some level and now was the time to address this. I spent the following two years doing online guided meditations every day. There are literally hundreds free on YouTube. These served many purposes; they trained me to relax deeply, they helped me address issues of inadequacy, to look deeply at my relationships with my parents and to understand where my feelings of inadequacy may have come from. My mother loved being pregnant and having babies but soon became more interested in the next pregnancy and baby. The hormonal changes during pregnancy may have temporarily soothed her depression, which she suffered from most of her life (I didn't realise this when I was small. Our home life was the only thing we knew and was therefore 'normal'. It was only much later, and especially since her death and reflecting on her life that I came to realise how unhappy she was for much of the time).

After the age of two or three, I got little attention or approval from either parent as my father just wasn't at home much. This, I believe, was the primary source of my low self-esteem. It certainly didn't help me in my choice of men until I was lucky enough to meet my wonderful husband in my early forties.

Louise Hay has some excellent meditations (free on YouTube) in which the aim is to forgive both your parents and yourself. My parents were doing the best they could with the tools at their disposal at the time. My mum, especially, had a difficult time as a very young child during the second world war. Her father was away at war and the small family had literally no money. Food was scarce, and the poverty they suffered is difficult to imagine in these affluent times. As a single example, one year they managed to get hold of a sheep's head for Christmas dinner, supposedly the best dinner of the year! When my grandad finally came back from the war, he had changed from an affable village grocer into a dark and somber personality, occasionally violent towards his wife. There are shocking family tales, which it would not be appropriate to go into here.

Over time I have come to terms with my parents and my past and am at peace with it all. It took a lot of work. I can sit still and relax now, without fidgeting. I will no longer do things I don't want to do, in order to try and please others or fulfil perceived obligations. I have learned how to say 'no' when I want to. In short, I have learned to love myself!

These days I take care to spend some time looking after myself every single day. I have read the inspirational work of Dr Joe Dispenza (especially Breaking the Habit of Being Yourself and Becoming Supernatural) which made me realise how much of my time was spent rerunning loops of negative past events in my mind, thus triggering stress hormones and preventing my body from resting and healing. (The body doesn't know the difference between what is going on in your head and what is occurring in the real world; it reacts in exactly the same way.) I now focus much more on the present moment and stay ever more alert to 'negative reruns' which I then consciously switch off. This takes work and practice and seems impossible at first.

Trust me, it IS possible and like any skill, improves with practice. I'm definitely still a work in progress.

Then there is the wonderful Dr Bruce Lipton with his book 'Biology of Belief'. His main message, as I understand it, is that your cells will listen to you. So it is vitally important to be mindful of the messages you send them. If you are convinced you are going to die, then in all likelihood you will. If you send positive messages about vibrant health and feeling great with a happy future ahead of you, then your cells will sit up and take notice of that too.

A body that moves frequently is generally healthier than a sedentary one. This I have tackled by doing plenty of brisk walking, out in nature whenever I can. I am also a keen cyclist although road cycling frightens me because I feel so vulnerable to the carelessness of others. In the UK in particular, there is a discernible dislike of cyclists. The continent is much better in this regard. In any event, I stick to mountain biking, which is really off-road cycling down various tracks and trails (no mountains involved!), again in nature as much as ever possible. I have also started the 'Couch to 5k' challenge (just completed week 1 of 9!). I have never been a runner but would very much like to run with relative ease for half an hour or so. I have no plans to run a marathon, but at 62 years of age, I am aware that muscle mass will diminish as time goes on and that exercising regularly will help to keep that to a minimum, as well as keeping blood and lymph circulating nicely and generally keeping things in good working order.

Use it or lose it as they say!

The most important physical activity I undertake is Qi Gong. I used to do yoga but came to realise that I will never be very flexible. I find Qi Gong much more holistic and look forward to it every day. I don't like to miss a day if I can help it. It consists of mostly gentle movements, linked with breath and visualization and helps to clear fixed and stuck energy in a similar way to acupuncture. It is also brilliant to help keep joints, fascia, tendons and ligaments strong and flexible. It vastly improves proprioception, a delightful word which means 'perception or awareness of the position and movement of the body'. Last but by no means not least, it helps calm stress levels in an almost miraculous way. I use free YouTube videos, especially those of Nick Loffree, a very talented young man who teaches beautifully, having brought himself back from the brink of a disastrous life featuring addiction and mental health problems.

Respect!

I would just mention briefly that I have a very small income and have little money to spare on expensive treatments. Over the years I have spent maybe two or three thousand pounds on supplements as and when the budget stretched to them. I have never visited any naturopaths or expensive private clinics. In a way I would love that, being cared for professionally in ways that go far beyond traditional oncology. It is simply beyond my means though, and up to now I love being in charge of my own destiny and decisions. Spending a fortune is not compulsory and I firmly believe true healing comes from within.

So this is where I'm at. Calm, healthy, enjoying every single day to the best of my ability and generally loving life. I don't think I would go so far as to say I'm glad I have had cancer but it has certainly woken me up to paths in life that I never dreamed of. It has taught me to love, care for, and respect myself and to treasure life and love above all other things. They really are the only things of any importance at all! Will I remain healthy? Who knows? I certainly intend to and will continue to work in that direction but beyond that, it's not really my concern. I have looked death squarely in the face and am not afraid of it. It will come eventually by one means or another. In the meantime, I am busy living my best life and planning for a happy and healthy old age.

If you are reading this, it is likely that you or a loved one is facing a cancer diagnosis. It is terrifying and feels like everything is spiraling out of control in a very bad way. Have a look at 'Radical Remission' (the book and the website). It is full of stories of people overcoming dire diagnoses and applying themselves to life with every fibre of their being, in all sorts of different ways, many of them with huge success. Take the time to check out some of Dr Joe Dispenza's YouTube videos in which people with cancer, many of them stage 4, and a variety of other health issues, tell their stories of success. Not all of them have paid a lot of money to attend his retreats! As Dr Joe says, surviving and thriving with cancer is like the four-minute mile. It seems impossible until somebody does it. As more and more people achieve it, it becomes ever more attainable to ordinary people like you and me.

I wish you every success.

Vanessa's Story

I woke up in a hospital bed. All I could think of was that I had to get my 23-month-old daughter; she had to be with me. Where was she? She'd never been apart from me. Maybe I could just have her stay right beside me in the hospital bed.

"Do you know where you are?" asked a nurse.

Still groggy from the anesthesia, I could guess I was at the hospital, but I did not realize I had been transferred to the largest hospital on Vancouver Island, the one with a neurosurgery ward.

Late the night before I had blacked out and fallen unconscious. I was unable to control my bodily functions. My idiotic boyfriend simply thought I had either COVID or food poisoning and left me alone in bed for *the entire night*. It was morning before he had the sense to call 911.

Following several weeks of intense tension headaches (which my doctor said was just due to low iron: *"take some iron supplements and follow up with me in a few months"*, he said), my brain tumor took over and threatened to end my life then and there.

Thankfully I held out through the night, and the hospital had more sense than my boyfriend (whose delayed reaction could very likely have killed me). They ran a CAT scan since I was too unstable to be put in the MRI machine. The neurosurgeon did not even have a clear picture of what he was up against, but miraculously, was able to perform a near-total resection of my brain tumor, which was roughly the size of a tennis ball, around 6-7cm, and located in my right temporal lobe.

While lying in the hospital bed after the surgery, the anesthesiologist dropped by to tell me what a remarkable recovery I had made, considering the shape I had been in when I arrived the day before.

The following day the surgeon came in to discuss the craniotomy. He said the pathology report would confirm the findings, but said the tumor was very likely cancerous, and probably a *Glioblastoma*.

I was incredulous when he said that the standard course of treatment would be chemotherapy and 6 weeks of radiation. "*6 weeks?*" I spat. It could not be possible. I had a baby. I was trying to leave an abusive relationship. I was exhausted, at the end of my rope. I was in no shape to battle cancer. But I quickly recovered from the surgery, and what should have been up to a 2-week hospital stay ended up being 5 short days. I was discharged with no deficits, no complications, no medications. I could walk, talk, see, speak, and eat just as though nothing had ever happened to me. I came home to my baby and my parents, who thankfully came over to help out.

5 days after falling into a coma, I was now a 30-something-year old new mom with a tennis-ball-sized hole in my brain, a cancer diagnosis with a grim prognosis, and very little strength. All I could do was recover. And fight.

Back home, grateful to be with my daughter, but crying every night about what was to come, many arrangements had to be made. In the span of a week, my life had turned upside down. But on the upside, my boyfriend finally left, and my parents took me and my daughter in to help me through my treatment. Moving back to my hometown with my parents was a necessary step, as it meant being much closer to the cancer center where I would get my treatment, plus having my mom look after my daughter.

And so began a year of appointments, MRIs, blood tests, chemotherapy pills, and radiation sessions. When I wasn't doing those things, I was desperately trying to do my own research to see what else could be done to avoid what seemed like the inevitable grim prognosis with glioblastoma (GBM): eventual tumor regrowth. I read that many people don't survive more than a year or two after the diagnosis. I was told the tumor was removed but that microscopic cancer cells remained. These cancer cells, being aggressive as this is a stage 4 cancer, would likely start to grow into another tumor.

The Cancer Agency led me through their standard of care treatment. My radiation treatments were 5 days a week for 6 weeks. They kept a close eye on me, but I hated being there. Not that anyone enjoys it. But it was all just too much sometimes. It was a full-time job. And I already had a full-time job, being a mom.

Thank goodness for my mom who was able to watch my daughter while I was getting the treatments. And thank goodness I was able to take the chemo pills at home, at bedtime every night, rather than have IV chemo like some people do. But it was still too much. I was sleep deprived and mentally exhausted. But I would be kept at the Cancer Agency for a checkup or a follow up, and sometimes it would take so long.

One nurse started questioning me, what was going on, why did I seem so anxious? I broke down in tears because I just wanted it all to stop. She suggested I make an appointment with a counselor at the cancer agency. Based on their cold, impersonal attitudes I just did not want to get counseling there. They all seemed so busy, so rushed and overworked. And I just felt like one of the hundreds upon thousands of cancer patients they see and treat each day. One of the herd.

Take your chemo, don't ask questions.

So, they upset me and then tell me I need counseling. I told them I have no appetite and am losing weight; they suggested I take dexamethasone, a powerful steroid that can actually trigger tumor regrowth. Thankfully I knew better and threw the prescription away.

Take steroids to help me eat more! Worst advice ever. At that point I completely lost faith in them.

My oncologist is a man of very few words with a terrible bedside manner. Even now after over 3 years of seeing him we have no rapport. My experience with the cancer agency has just been get in, get out, and forget about it. I did my 6 weeks of radiation and concurrent chemotherapy (Temodar/Temozolomide). I continued chemo, doing it for a full 12 months. Now I return to see my oncologist twice a year for a brief follow-up appointment to discuss my MRI results. Every 5-6 months I have MRI imaging done to monitor and check for any recurrence. To my relief, every single MRI has come back stable, with no signs of tumor regrowth.

I do not believe this standard of care alone is what brought me to where I am today, over 3 years past my surgery. I think it only bought me time. Am I glad I did it? Sure. Because I had to try everything. And SOC was not enough. So here's what else I did.

Before I get into the complementary approaches I used, I'd like to mention my prognosis. Initially, I did not want to know what it was, but I found out about it when my mom and I got into a fight one day. It was about some petty things like the dishes or who was using the kitchen (I was living with my parents while doing SOC and while I really had no choice but to stay with them, it was also really, really tough).

I remember yelling to my mom "I'm dying of cancer!" and her response was…"Oh. Well, no you're not; the doctor said you had 3-5 years!"….and I was just so shocked and dumbfounded that she would be tactless enough to tell me my prognosis; obviously nobody had told her I didn't wish to know! So now I have to go forward knowing I only have 3-5 years to live, according to the cancer agency. I've since learned to ignore the prognosis, and completely put these numbers out of my head.

Much of what I learned about integrative cancer treatments I found online, through glioblastoma communities, and from other long-term GBM survivors. It was recommended that I start a protocol of off-label prescription medications. These are commonly used medications which can be repurposed and taken for their anti-tumour and cancer stem-cell-destroying properties.

Of course, there was little chance an ordinary MD would prescribe these, so I was lucky to be able to find a doctor in the U.S. who was happy to send me the medications. For about 2 ½ years now I have been taking about 8 different off-label medications; my "GBM cocktail" if you will, which I believe has really helped to stop any tumor regrowth. From metformin, a diabetes medication which regulates blood sugar, to doxycycline, an antibiotic which can kill cancer stem cells, this daily regime took up a lot of my time. In addition to this I started consulting with a master herbalist/nutritionist also based out of the US, who continues to advise me on which supplements to take as well as helpful dietary choices to make.

Initially she had me take supplements which would complement my chemo/radiation and help them work better - such as curcumin and artemisia. Of course, try telling my oncologist or radiologist I was taking these, and they would not have been happy. So it was an unwritten don't ask, don't tell policy between us. They continue to have no idea what supplements and medications I take.

I really believe that the supplements helped me to get through SOC and to maintain my health following surgery. They also helped to finally get my blood count back up to stable levels, 3 years after completing SOC.

It's hard to keep track of everything I tried in my cancer battle. I also took THC and CBD oils to help fight a recurrence and generally to help keep nausea at bay during SOC, so I was able to eat. I took essiac tea before bed as this combination of herbs such as sheep sorrel is said to help with cancer. And last but not least, I had a series of personal peptide vaccines made for me (9 vaccines to be exact) which my naturopath administered over a 6 month period. These peptides are part of a more recent approach to cancer fighting called immunotherapy. Although seen as experimental, it is gaining more ground and becoming more recognized. The vaccines I took are now part of a US clinical trial, and there are others available of a similar nature.

In a nutshell, that has been my journey with GBM. It's been over 3 years and I am feeling better than I have in years. I'm not only surviving; I'm thriving. Although I lost about 20 pounds during chemo, I gained the weight back. I am sleeping better than I have in years and am overall feeling alright.

Oncology has really played only a minimal role in helping me stay NED (*no evidence of disease*). I feel that carving out my own cancer healing journey while keeping a positive attitude has done wonders for my wellbeing, moreso than any oncological intervention.

I would have to say that I cannot pinpoint just *one* type of treatment that has helped me to stay alive. I firmly believe that everything has helped me in my healing journey. I know SOC does not work for everyone, but I do think that chemo and radiation helped *along with* the supplements, off label medications, and the peptide vaccine.

It's just that relying on oncology alone is not enough. The fact that they are so one-sided as opposed to holistic in their treatment approach does not help.

It is beyond belief that cancer centers are not more holistic, or at least mine isn't. There's no focus on diet, psychology, mental health, but rather a very limited reliance on chemo and radiation. I think that's why so many cancer patients have poor outcomes. One would think that in 2023 oncology would "wake up" and begin to embrace complementary and integrative approaches to cancer treatment, but it seems to have stuck its head in the sand and refuses to budge. I am hopeful that stories of long-term cancer survivors will influence and empower others to expand their cancer-treating horizons and to embrace a multi-faceted approach to cancer treatment and care.

. . .

Diagnosis in April 2020: *Glioblastoma multiforme* (GBM)

Completed 6 months of radiation and one year of chemotherapy in 2020.

Received 9 personal peptide vaccines in 2021.

3 years later: surviving and thriving with no deficits, complications, or recurrences. Every MRI has come back stable with no signs of tumor regrowth.

Ann's Story, Part 4

My only option to continue chemotherapy was to make the trek to Stanford. By now, it was almost December. The mountain passes were closed and the weather dicey.

My husband had badly needed knee replacement surgery scheduled for 12/21/22, which meant I had to be at the top of my game to take care of the household and snow removal. Schlepping back and forth to Stanford for weekly Taxol infusions just wasn't in the cards.

I had my initial phone consultation with Sean Devlin, DO, an integrative oncologist also boarded in family medicine. He was pleasant, professional, personable. My visit with him was right after I'd discovered the infusion center had dumped me. Dr. Devlin was kind and supportive, something I truly needed in that moment.

Over the next few months, we talked several times. He ordered CARIS genomic testing right off the bat.

Lo and behold, CARIS is a mainstream test. So mainstream, Medicare paid for it. Kaiser uses it to sort out who will (and won't) benefit from chemotherapy. They've always been pioneers in terms of making the best use of resources.

My results were interesting. The way the test works is CARIS gets a tissue sample from your tumor. Pathology departments keep things like that for a period of time, and at that point I was less than a year out from my original surgery.

According to my tumor genomics, chemotherapy never would have helped me.

This bears repeating.

The poison four oncologists (five if you count the one from Sutter) were willing to fall on their swords for, never would have helped me. All it would have done was trash my immune system.

I'm told I was an outlier, but I wonder how true that is.

The Stanford MD had the good grace to apologize because this type of testing wasn't yet on Stanford's radar. She further said to not let anyone give me any more chemo.

According to my CARIS results, if I do get a recurrence, an immunotherapy is indicated. The test also reassured me I didn't have any of the "bad" genes like BRCA or KRAS, and that my tumor mutational burden was quite low. That can cut both ways in that it may mean immunotherapy wouldn't work for me, either. Hard to say. Last time I looked up tumor mutational burden, there was new research indicating it being low was positive prognostically.

Cancer is complex and a rapidly shifting field.

By now, in my opinion Dr. Devlin had been elevated to godhood. He, a humble family medicine boarded physician (who also did a four-year integrative oncology fellowship and has several Ph.D.s), knew more about how to proceed than board certified oncologists.

I stopped bemoaning only having had two chemo infusions and decided the goddess was looking out for me. Working as a team, Dr. Devlin and I came up with every other week intravenous vitamin C infusions preceded by artesunate. I did that for a year.

In case anyone is wondering about radiation, there is solid research out there that clearly proves radiation doesn't alter outcomes for my type of cancer. Despite that, both the gyn onc surgeons from my original surgeries, and the gal I saw at Sutter Health, all pushed for it.

Once I had that second surgery, the Stanford MD was quite clear my urinary system was far too fragile for radiation. And she did tell me it didn't matter because radiation wouldn't alter outcomes. My question is why so many gyn oncs still push radiation. It has big downsides including development of other cancers years down the road.

Backtracking to the winter of 21-22. It was difficult. My husband's surgery happened, and we had a ten-day storm immediately afterward. I spent the next three weeks outside shoveling snow multiple times a day. I was still depleted from the chemo I'd had, but I was out there anyway doing what I had to do to keep our household together.

No one who hasn't lived in a place like Mammoth Lakes truly appreciates what it takes to deal with hundreds of inches of snow that just keep on falling. You survive by not getting too far ahead of the curve. I'm convinced all that backbreaking labor was good for me and killed off any remaining cancer cells.

Intense physical exercise creates an environment that is incompatible for circulating tumor cells and cancer stem cells (CSCs).

Since I brought CSCs up, let's spend a bit of time discussing them. Chemotherapy can make CSCs stronger and more resilient. They are not fast-growing cells, so chemo doesn't touch them, but they are a big reason why people get recurrences.

The following is excerpted from Targeting Cancer Stem Cell Pathways for Cancer Therapy by Yang, et al. in the journal Signal Transduction and Targeted Therapy 2/07/2020.

"The main reasons for the failure of cancer treatment are metastasis, recurrence, heterogeneity, resistance to chemotherapy and radiotherapy, and avoidance of immunological surveillance. All these failures could be explained by the characteristics of cancer stem cells (CSCs). CSCs can cause cancer recurrence, metastasis, multidrug resistance, and radiation resistance through their ability to arrest in the G0 phase, giving rise to new tumors. (The G0 phase is a resting phase where the cell has left the cycle and stopped dividing.)

Therefore, CSCs could be considered the most promising targets for cancer treatment."

An important point is traditional chemotherapy and radiotherapy make CSCs more resistant to eradication. So the treatments that are supposed to cure us merely kick the can down the road. It also means you don't get a second chance to pick the right agent for first-line treatment. The only way you manage that is by doing some type of genomic/molecular testing first.

Before you have any treatment at all, it's important to know ahead of time if the agent the MD has chosen has a prayer of being effective against your specific cancer. As we've established, Robert Nagourney MD heads up the Nagourney Cancer Institute in Long Beach, California. He pioneered using fresh tumor samples to determine what actually kills them. Sometimes, it isn't the "standard of care" recommended drug.

Once you've taken that SOC drug, however, you've lessened the odds of the proper agent working if/when you finally get around to it.

A bit more about CSCs (also from the Yang, et al, article) and how critical they are to the field of cancer treatment follows. Interestingly, they are largely ignored by most oncologists who adhere to a standard of care model.

Biological characteristics of CSCs

"With the deepening of tumor biology research, clinical diagnosis and cancer treatment have significantly improved in recent years. However, the high recurrence rate and high mortality rate are still unresolved and are closely related to the biological characteristics of CSCs. With further understanding of CSC characteristics, research on tumor biology has entered a new era. Therefore, understanding the biological properties of CSCs is of great significance in the diagnosis and treatment of tumors.

"CSCs have a strong self-renewal ability, which is the direct cause of tumorigenesis. CSCs can symmetrically divide into two CSCs or into one CSC and one daughter cell. CSCs expand in a symmetrical splitting manner to excessively increase cell growth, ultimately leading to tumor formation. CSCs isolated from original tumor tissue that were transplanted into severe combined immunodeficiency disease (SCID) mice then formed new tumors.

"It is currently believed that CSCs are the key "seeds" for tumor initiation and development, metastasis, and recurrence. CSCs have evolved and are highly heterogeneous. The heterogeneity of CSCs has also been found in other cancers, including glioblastoma, prostate cancer, and lung cancer. The heterogeneity of CSCs is so complex that more effective biomarkers are needed to identify CSCs or distinguish their heterogeneity."

Apologies. That was a lot of pretty heavy science. The take-home message is cancer stem cells are implicated in most (if not all) recurrences. Being given an incorrect chemotherapeutic agent can empower CSCs and make further treatment less efficacious.

My bully pulpit, garnered from my particular experiences, is you have to ask questions. I believe everyone diagnosed with cancer needs genomic/molecular testing to determine the most promising course of treatment. I further believe this testing needs to occur BEFORE any treatment beyond surgery happens. We have the tools to enhance survivability. We should use them.

Let's segue into another survivor story or two.

Eleanor Hall's Story

In 2015, I experienced abdominal bloating. My GP said, maybe it's lactose intolerance. I cut out dairy products and that didn't help. I didn't pursue it because the bloating was only mildly uncomfortable.

Then I saw online that bloating and weight loss were symptoms of ovarian cancer. I had lost around nine pounds without trying to lose weight. I told my doctor and a mass in my abdomen was identified. Surgery in May, 2016 showed it was Stage IIIC ovarian cancer, pulmonary type, a rare type in which the cells are like lung cancer cells. My surgeon said that chemo would be of little or no help and I was eligible for hospice!

Fortunately, I got a second opinion at U. of Chicago Medicine. My doctor said I couldn't be cured but my life could be prolonged, she couldn't say how long. Although 80 years old, I was living an interesting, useful and active life, working on climate issues and a member of the board of my condo. I said, "I want to live."

I did not feel anxious or depressed. Rather, I simply wanted to do all I could to prolong my life.

Then, I had chemotherapy (**Carboplatin** and **etoposide**) and radiation therapy. I also consulted two Traditional Chinese Medicine practitioners. I was fortunate in that I have a cousin who is a TCM practitioner, Jonathan Hadas Edwards, living in North Carolina. Therefore, I was aware of it and sought out a TCM practitioner **in Chicago** recommended by my cousins' **colleagues**, Stephen Bonzak. I also consulted Kenji Aoki, a TCM practitioner in my neighborhood who was recommended by a friend. Bonzak prescribed herbs; Aoki prescribed black (roasted) garlic, which WebMD says fights some cancers.[1] I started TCM treatment right after my surgery, about the same time I started my chemo. (Unfortunately, many cancer patients don't seek out alternative treatments until western medicine has failed them.) I checked out the herbs and black garlic prescribed by the TCM practitioners with my oncologist. She had no problem with them.

I also made an effort to eat the foods on a cancer-fighting list I got from a workshop at University of Chicago Medicine. Web MD has a similar list. Cancer-fighting foods include blueberries, cruciferous vegetables, cherries, dark green leafy vegetables, green tea, soy, walnuts, black garlic, and others.

The only side effects from the chemo were fatigue and hair loss. I know some women buy wigs. But they are expensive and it didn't seem worth it, since I knew my

hair would grow back before long. So instead of a wig, I bought two caps offered by Tender Loving Care, under the American Cancer Society (https://www.tlcdirect.org). A friend also knitted a charcoal gray cap for me. All were becoming and worked well.

Now, six years after surgery, I have no evidence of cancer! One of my University of Chicago doctors said I had done remarkably well. I feel very fortunate. Many women in my situation would not have survived.

I know that ovarian cancer is called the silent killer because so often it is diagnosed too late to be cured. Has any research been done on why some women are diagnosed at Stage I or II, others at Stage III or IV? I haven't read of any. I asked my GP about my diagnosis and he said, bloating has many causes and my weight loss wasn't that great from one visit to the next. But when I mentioned my abdominal bloating, he could have said, "It may be lactose intolerance. Try cutting out dairy products. If that doesn't help, let me know." If I had gone back to him sooner, I would have been diagnosed earlier.

A journal article, a case report, has been written about me.[2] In the first draft, TCM was not mentioned. I said it should be included. It was added, but in the body of the article. In the conclusions, all the credit was given to the chemo and the radiation therapy. I do think that the chemo was important in my cure. In a journal article I read, my kinds of chemo were more effective than several other kinds of chemo that have been used on my kind of cancer. But I also think the Traditional Chinese Medicine contributed. The same journal article said that the majority of patients with my kind of cancer don't survive more than a year or two. My kind of cancer is so rare that a major study on treatment will never be done. The best treatment will only be arrived at through case reports like mine on the effects of different kinds of treatment. So I am glad to have contributed to the medical knowledge on ovarian cancer.

Sharon Ann Merritt's Story

On April 2018, I was diagnosed with HER2+ breast cancer, after having a mammogram because of a nipple discharge. HER2+ (positive) breast cancer is when breast cancer cells have excessive amounts of a protein receptor called HER2 (human epidermal growth factor receptor 2). Normally, this protein helps breast cells grow, divide, and repair themselves. But sometimes, something goes wrong in the gene that controls the HER2 protein and the breast cells make too many of these receptors. This causes your breast cells to grow and divide uncontrollably, causing breast cancer. About 1 of 5 breast cancers are HER2+.

I was rushed through the traditional protocol, MRI, and surgeon appointment. The surgeon's recommendation was immediate lumpectomy and radiation. When I informed the surgeon I wanted to think about it, he informed me I had no time to wait, or I would also need chemo. Fortunately, two friends stopped me from going the traditional route and sent me off on a holistic journey. One of them was an oncology nurse who had healed her breast cancer herself. She gave me books to read and supplements to take. From there I researched everything I could and threw it at the cancer. I also did and continue to do extensive psychotherapy, including EMDR, to deal with past trauma as there is an emotional link to breast cancer.

Fast forward to July 2020, I heard about a blood biopsy done in Greece that could predict the supplements that would kill your specific cancer. I found a group on Facebook and a lady that recommended a doctor in Irvine, CA. I made an appointment and had the test done. At my follow up visit in August with Dr. Connealy, she suggested I research cryoablation. I joined a Facebook group where Jennifer Pinto told me about a surgeon in Glendale, CA, Dr. Dennis Holmes. I sent him all my records and he accepted me as a patient "off protocol" (which means that I'm not a part of a study and needed to pay up front). His assistant set up a consult. At the consultation, he said he suspected my nipple and areolar skin changes were Paget's disease of the breast and recommended a biopsy. I had seen several doctors for the nipple, and he was the only one who recognized the Paget's. The others told me they were pretty sure it wasn't since it's supposedly rare. I was already sure after lots of research it was Paget's, so I didn't need a biopsy. I just asked him to remove it, and he agreed.

On Sept 30, 2020, I arrived at Dr. Holmes's office for cryoablation and to have the Paget's nipple removed. Being as meticulous as he is, he first did his own ultrasound and found a second tumor that was missed by 5 radiologists on the previous scans. He proceeded to numb the breast and do a biopsy of the newly discovered tumor. He made a very small incision and then using a Cryoprobe (a needle-like instrument through which liquid nitrogen circulates to treat cancer by freezing it until it is dead), he froze the first tumor. The freezing lasted about 8 minutes followed by a 10-minute thaw phase followed again by another 8 minutes of freezing. The freeze zone extends approximately 5-10 mm beyond the tumor to allow for clean margins. The freeze/thaw cycle injures the cancer cells, killing them. He then removed the nipple and placed it in a container to be sent to pathology. Once the stitching of the wound was done, Dr. Holmes proceeded to freeze the second tumor. The whole procedure took about two-and-a-half hours due to two tumors and the minor surgery. All done in his office. It was amazing. A simple tiny incision vs. a scar and no significant recovery time. The only side effects were swelling from the saline injected to protect the skin from the freeze and a lump of dead tissue. The swelling dissipated in a few weeks. The lump continues to dissolve over time. I was fortunate to not have any bruising, which is not typical. I left the office with a dressing on my incision from the nipple removal and a Band-Aid on the incision where the Cryoprobe was inserted. We drove the almost two hours home, and I made dinner. The next day I went back to my normal activities.

The biopsy of the second tumor also came back HER2+. The nipple biopsy came back Paget's, as I expected. Following Dr. Holmes's recommendation, I did 6-months of Herceptin infusions to kill any HER2+ breast cancer cells remaining in my body.

Three months later, Dr. Holmes did a follow up ultrasound that showed no evidence of disease. At six months I had an MRI, ultrasound, and biopsy. MRI and ultrasound were clear, and the biopsy came back benign, no malignancy. A year later I couldn't feel the mass.

I was recently privileged to observe Dr. Holmes perform a cryoablation procedure. It is amazing to see how a simple in-office procedure can replace lumpectomy or mastectomy for some breast cancer patients. Losing a women's breast is a very traumatic experience. Avoiding the loss of a breast would save a lot of grief for women who have the option. Of course, for some cryoablation is not an option. But for those who could have the option, it should be made available. Not only does it prevent a lot of trauma and pain, but it is also extremely cost-effective. If insurance covered cryoablation they would be paying out a lot less than what they pay for the lumpectomies and mastectomies with reconstruction. I feel so blessed to have been given the option of cryoablation and to have the most caring, compassionate, and brilliant surgeon—Dr. Dennis Holmes. I will be forever grateful to him.

Unfortunately, doctors are not able to accept insurance for cryoablation because a reimbursement value has yet to be established for the cryoablation billing code (0581T). Furthermore, the billing code only covers one freezing/cryoablation, and many times more than one is required for larger cancers. That's if the insurance covers it at all. Most insurance companies are still considering it experimental even though it's been done successfully for over 12 years in the U.S. In my case I had two tumors which required two freezings/cryoablations, but Medicare only covered one. However, I was able to self-bill Medicare after the procedure using their Patient's Request for Medical Payment form. I filled out the form and included my doctor's receipt for services and procedure notes from the doctor. I was glad to see that at least I was reimbursed 80% of the cost of one tumor which in my case was about 50% of my total cost.

For private insurance I would recommend doing the same as I did for Medicare. All insurance companies have an out-of-network patient request-for-payment form. File that form with the doctor's receipt for services and the procedure notes. If the claim is denied, file an appeal. If they deny the appeal, then contact the insurance company's customer service and ask who has jurisdiction over the insurance company. Then file an appeal with that jurisdiction. In that appeal you could say that, if Medicare approves and pays for this procedure, then private insurance should as well. The jurisdiction can override the insurance companies' denial and force them to pay. I've had success doing that in the past with other issues. We need to fight the system until cryoablation becomes standard of care for breast cancer. It's time that insurance companies covered cryoablation for breast cancer just as they do for other cancers (including prostate cancer). You can also use a third-party biller (a professional biller who bills the insurance on your behalf) to bill the insurance. I know ladies that belong to medical coops get their cryoablation covered and others who have managed to get some insurance coverage.

I also want to say how much I appreciate Dr. Dennis Holmes. His passion for helping breast cancer patients is contagious. My life has been forever changed because of meeting him. I have learned so much from him and want to share my knowledge with other ladies. Together, Dr. Holmes and I raised $30,000 for a clinical trial for Cryoablation of DCIS with the help of Doterra Healing Hands Foundation Matching program. Dr. Holmes is currently recruiting for this trial.

It has now become my ministry to advocate for cryoablation, Dr. Holmes, and the many women who can benefit from this procedure. In the year since I had my cryoablation I have had the privilege of sharing with many other ladies who have now also been spared surgery through cryoablation. I spend countless hours on Facebook getting the word out and supporting the ladies no matter which journey they chose. It's important that ladies know all their choices and make their own informed decision when facing a breast cancer or DCIS diagnosis. Doctors should present all possible options, make their recommendations, and then respect the ladies' right to choose what they are comfortable with, not dictate what they "have" to do. After all, the ladies are the ones that must live with the decision and the outcome, not the doctor. I have been very blessed with a team of doctors that educate me on all my options, let me do my research, and then respect my choices, even if they disagree. It wasn't easy to find my doctors. I fired a few along the way. Cancer is stressful enough on its own. It's important to have supportive doctors whom you respect and who respect you. It's also extremely important that you do your own research. Don't be afraid to ask questions. If a doctor doesn't want to answer your questions, find one who will. Take one day at a time and breathe. You can get through this!

It's my hope and prayer cryoablation for breast cancer will soon become part of the standard of care, be covered by all insurance, and not be limited to covering only one freezing.

In July 2021 Dr. Holmes surprised me by asking me if I would interview him for his upcoming webinar. Of course, I said yes. I was flattered he asked me after sending out a notice saying he had a special guest coming to interview him. It was just the beginning. Three months later he asked me to do an encore. Going forward we do these webinars almost every other month. I collect questions from cancer patients they would like Dr. Holmes to answer. It gives a place for patients to ask questions they may be afraid to ask their surgeon, or maybe they want to hear another perspective. I have learned so much myself doing these webinars and totally enjoy doing them.

In February 2022 Dr. Holmes asked me, to my surprise, if I would like to partner with him in a new business creating products to make recovery from surgery easier for patients. I spent the next year developing a cape for patients to use so they could take a shower right after surgery. Surgery is traumatic enough without being told you can't take a shower. This product can be found at https://recovereasy.com.

In March 10, 2022, I met Dr. Maggie Gama for the first time She was a Godsend. She's my primary care doctor. She's integrative and many of her patients are cancer patients. She has helped me so much in getting my immune system and body on the right track. And she takes insurance. I feel so blessed.

In November 2022 I was having some shoulder pain. I asked my masseur, Tony, to work on it. He suggested I also get my chiropractor to adjust it. So, my Chiropractor, Derek, suggested I get an abdominal ultrasound to see if maybe I had a gallstone. Dr. Gama ordered the ultrasound. I was shocked by the results. I did have a gallstone, but I also had a 4 cm spot on my liver. Dr. Holmes and Dr. Gama became my biggest advocates after my oncologist told me I wasn't curable anymore, and said she knew it was going to happen. She didn't approve of my other doctors.

I was devastated. I didn't need that negativity. I told Dr. Holmes about my experience with her, and his response was, "It's manageable. We just must find you the right treatment."

He literally peeled me off the wall, and at midnight no less. It was Thanksgiving week, and he ordered a CT, PET/CT, bone scan, brain scan, and a liver biopsy. All were done before Christmas. He then got me an appointment with his friend, Linnea Chap MD, a breast cancer only medical oncologist.

She was awesome. Rather than tell me it was bad, she told me she had a patient who has been on Herceptin for over 20 years and is doing great. She didn't make any promises, but she gave me hope. By January 10 she had me in treatment. She was good about listening to my concerns. I really didn't want to lose my hair. At first, she talked about Taxol but changed it to Xeloda, a chemo pill. Given she is about a 3-hour drive from my house it was a better alternative than having to make the trip every day for weeks. She wanted me to do three 500mg pills twice a day, but I asked for a reduced dose and we went with two twice a day, one week, one week off. Also, Herceptin and Perjeta infusions every three weeks. Within three weeks, my liver enzymes were normal. By the end of February, the liver metastasis wasn't active, and by the end of April it was completely resolved.

May 9 I was finished with Xeloda. I had minimal side effects. I will continue Herceptin and Perjeta indefinitely. I continue with IV vitamin C and IV ozone to keep my immune system in good shape as well as massage and chiropractic weekly. Dr. Gama and Dr. Chap have been my other great advocates. Dr. Gama has been totally supportive of Dr. Chap's choice of treatment. I love having all my doctors on the same page. It gives me great comfort that I will be okay. I do want to emphasize though that my choice to have cryoablation had nothing to do with my progressing to stage 4. Cryoablation replaces surgery. Her2 is very aggressive and had probably advanced to my liver prior to the cryoablation and we just didn't know it. Distant metastasis of Her2+ positive breast cancer are known to progress from invisible to detectable in 2-3 years, especially when treated without anti-Her2 therapy, which I had initially declined. My liver metastasis took a little over 2 years to appear.

In April my husband and I went to Las Vegas with Dr. Holmes to display our capes at the NCoBC, national interdisciplinary breast cancer conference, and in May the three of us went to the American Society of Breast surgeons conference in Boston. I had no problem doing these trips while doing my treatments. Life has never been better. Cancer for me has been a blessing. I've met the most wonderful people, and I have an amazing team of doctors. I'm looking forward to a long, interesting, and fulfilling life.

I do travel almost two hours to do the webinars and three hours or more to Beverly Hills for my treatments but it's totally worth it to have the best doctors. I'll also be going to the Lynn Sage conference in Chicago in September as a Susan Komen science advocate for training. My life is so fulfilling now. I have a husband who goes to all my treatments with me and three daughters and seven grandkids. Life is good. I wish everyone could have doctors like I do, so supportive and positive. Live life like you don't have cancer while doing what you have to do to treat it.

Ann's note: Stories like these give me hope there are caring, compassionate oncologists in the world. Many thanks to Sharon for sharing hers.

Ann's Story, Part 5

We left off with me shoveling snow during the winter of 21-22.

One element I haven't mentioned is that, despite cold capping, I lost bunches of hair. I had bald spots and broken, badly damaged tresses. Round about the middle of April, I had it cut extremely short. I hated it, but at least it looked like a choice and didn't scream, "cancer survivor."

By now, I'd had a few more phone consults with Dr. Devlin. I already told you that we decided to try me on intravenous vitamin C (a high dose) preceded by artesunate. Dr. Devlin accomplished what the infusion center at the hospital in Bishop couldn't. He said I had to have a port, so in early March 2022 I went to an interventional radiologist in Reno and had one placed.

The whole procedure took maybe an hour, but I was sore and miserable for the next two months. In truth, I never truly got used to it. The insertion site always bothered me, and I felt it when I rolled over in bed. Backpacking was off the table because the pack pulled on the skin over the port.

Hefting shovelfuls of snow was miserable.

But the worst part was it served as a constant reminder I had cancer.

Healing has mental as well as physical components. Anxiety and stress are not your friends since cancer feeds on them. What I needed was breaks from the whole cancer gig. Times when I could just be normal.

It was tough since I was traveling to Reno every two weeks for infusions. They began toward the end of March 2022. Dr. Devlin wanted me to stay for two days and have IVC + artesunate two days running. It was a nice theory, but those trips north took two days as it was. Had I stayed an extra day, they'd have taken three. And the infusions were expensive. $1300 each trip, mostly because artesunate is pricey.

Two days would have run close to three grand, twice a month. That's $72,000 for a year. As it was, I spent well over $40,000.

All this was out of pocket. I finally got around to billing Medicare. They laughed at me, which was interesting since chemo would have cost them more by a factor of a hundred or so.

In addition to my biweekly treks north, I beefed up my supplement regimen. Maria Wessling Bachteal, whose story is included in this book, graciously agreed to consult with me despite me not having breast cancer.

She finetuned my supplements after mapping the pathways from mutations noted on my CARIS genomic testing.

I continued weekly acupuncture, weekly psychotherapy, my daily gratitude journal, twice daily meditation, intermittent fasting, rebound training, and a daily exercise/yoga/stretching program. I also did my best to watch my diet. Many cancer gurus push a whole food plant-based diet.

I tried. Honestly, I did, but weight simply sloughed off me. I've never been overweight, so I didn't have any leeway. After my third go round with whole food plant based (WFPB), I gave up and retreated to paleo, a proven eating plan that I can tolerate. And one that maintains my weight within about a five-pound window.

In case anyone is interested, intravenous Vitamin C isn't exactly a picnic. It crashes your blood sugar. I discovered early on it went better if I brought food and basically ate through the three hours I was getting infused.

During those months, I added to my cancer library. It was a rare week when I wasn't trolling through PubMed researching this, that, or the other. I bought books and inhaled them. The ones I found most important are listed toward the back of this book in the resource section.

My scans and bloodwork continued to be mostly normal with the exception of one kidney marker. My blood pressure went through the roof whenever I walked into a clinic, so much so I invested in a home cuff. It was quite the relief to discover my pressure was normal at home when I wasn't stressed.

I also purchased a glucometer at Dr. Devlin's direction and check my blood sugar often enough to know it sits around 75-80 when I get up in the morning and doesn't go over 110 two hours after a meal.

Despite the sugar-laden junk food at every infusion center in the U.S., sugar is not your friend if you have cancer. We've established that glucose is one of cancer's primary metabolic pathways, and it's in your best interest to keep it nice and low.

Diet is a hot-button topic.

I've noted the sugar connection on a Facebook group I belong to that's specific to my kind of cancer. This is not an integrative care group, and I've skirted being kicked out when I've mentioned things like genomic testing.

And sugar.

The pushback from other group members goes something like:

"My doctor said I can eat whatever I want."

"My doctor said the whole sugar thing is a myth."

"I drink every night. My MD said it's fine." (Alcohol metabolizes as sugar…)

"I asked my oncologist if my weight was a problem. He told me to keep on eating." (This was a woman who weighed over 300 pounds. Obesity is a significant risk factor for many cancers including gynecologic ones.)

My take on that is these doctors don't exactly care if their patients survive, let alone thrive. But I've kept my mouth shut.

Or perhaps it runs deeper than not caring. My bet is oncologists are tired. The one who fired me confided she'd chosen oncology because she figured it would be black and white. When she discovered mostly shades of gray, it distressed her.

Tired doctors (or tired anyone else) don't want to pick up the gauntlet and engage in battles they figure are a lost cause from the gate. Patient diet/weight falls under that rubric as does alcohol consumption.

The other hot potato is cachexia. It's a wasting syndrome that actually kills more cancer patients than cancer. So doctors figure eating anything is better than eating nothing.

"Whatever you do, don't lose weight."

Somewhere along the line, the well-proven link between obesity and cancer got lost in the shuffle.

This brings up something I'd like to highlight, though. If you ask ten oncologists about a specific issue, you'll like as not get at least eight different answers. There's little concordance in terms of "whole person" treatment. Very few are willing to think outside the box.

Dr. Nagourney labeled this tendency institutional denialism when I interviewed him.

Makes it tough for us, the end-point users, to determine what kind of care we're getting. For me, this highlights why we have to become our own advocates, do our own research, ask our own questions.

If your doctor (like some of mine) either refuses to answer, changes the subject, or fires you from their practice, find someone else. Obviously, you'd have to if you were dumped from practice but consider it a gift.

MDs who are so narrow minded and have such fragile egos they cannot deal with researching topics on your behalf don't deserve your time.

If you have cancer, your life is on the line.

Yours, not theirs.

They are the experts. They owe you either answers or an "I don't know, but I'll find out."

They work for you, not the other way round.

Backtracking to diet. Regardless of what you eat, you want to avoid foods that are inflammatory. What do I mean by that? Grain and dairy aren't great. Processed foods and sugar are dealbreakers. Protein sources should be grassfed or wild caught.

My next-door neighbor is a fifteen-year breast cancer survivor. She got lucky because her caregivers were forward thinking enough to stress intense aerobic exercise, acupuncture, and a diet that avoided grain, dairy, and sugar. This was back around 2008 at UCLA. She had extensive disease spread (23 of 30 lymph nodes were positive), and she's still here.

But she's careful to adhere to her anti-cancer diet. And she insisted on continuing her aromatase inhibitor (a type of estrogen blocker) when the MDs wanted her to quit.

Compare her with another friend of mine who also had breast cancer. Unlike my neighbor with her double mastectomy, this friend wanted a lumpectomy. She didn't alter her diet, and she stopped hormone blockers at the five-year mark. Two years later the cancer resurfaced. Three years after that, she was dead.

We all get cancer for a reason. Since we'll never know for sure exactly what it was, it makes sense to hedge your bets. If you change nothing, whatever created cancer in your body in the first place could strike again.

It's up to you, but very little in my life is worth going to the mat for. I made a lot of changes after my diagnosis because I want to live.

Cards serve as a metaphor. So long as you don't run out of cards, you get to keep playing. Piggybacking on that, you can up the odds of holding onto your cards if you watch what you eat, take supplements specific to your cancer and genomics, and get a lot of exercise.

Feeling a wee bit guilty as I type that since we're on a five-week road trip with the Winnebago. Those trips are hideous for both exercise and a decent diet, but I'll be home soon and can resurrect my daily structure.

On the plus side, road trips are good for my spirit. I meet new people and see many interesting things. Perhaps there's a balance point.

Let's do another survivor story and then take a good, hard look at integrative care clinics.

Lena Winslow's Story

"The oak fought the wind and was broken, the willow bent when it must and survived."— Robert Jordan, The Fires of Heaven

Self-advocacy cancer journey:

Diagnosis, treatment decision, post treatment.

Most people can remember the day of a cancer diagnosis with great detail. Emotionally it feels like a fork in the road, a turning point, a blast that comes out of nowhere and changes everything. For me it was a phone call. She said, "You have a little cancer."

My immediate reaction was, what do you mean "little"? There is no such thing as LITTLE cancer... I felt disconnected, anxious, shocked, fearful, and confused. My life flashed before my eyes, and I started crying as if to mourn my life. Mourn because I knew I could never get my old life back, my life just before those words were spoken. As part of this report I will be focusing on the emotional aspect of cancer while utilizing and expanding on 7 core areas of health and how I addressed each of them with myself.

Those areas are: Relationships, Resiliency, Spirituality, Movement, Nutrition, Sleep, Environment. Together these form a core for healing and maintaining health, and I used them continuously throughout my treatment and recovery. I chose this order because this was the focus of intensity order in my case. I also reviewed all 7 throughout the entire journey from diagnosis to treatment completion to survivorship integrating them into a lifestyle I live today.

Which are the most important? The ones I was NOT currently addressing. The work that I avoided is the work that I NEEDED to engage in the most. My most neglected core area was dealing with family trauma and its effect on my relationship to myself and others. I realized I am great at compartmentalizing and also that much of my struggles were rooted there.

Compartmentalization was no longer doing the job, and I was going to have to open some boxes. Working with this as a medical professional and a patient was tricky. Dr. Rhode told me after reviewing my audio submission that motivational interviewing with family members is very difficult to do. Here I was going to work on myself. I believe I was successful conducting an interview with my daughter because of the process of self-knowledge and advocacy I am about to describe.

Shortly after diagnosis I worked thru the book by Dr. Mark Wolynn (Wolynn, (2017) *It Didn't Start Within You*. Penguin Books). I knew the foundation of my relationship with myself and my support system lay within my ability to shine a spotlight on family trauma. Not unleashing all of it on myself in the midst of cancer treatment. I knew I had to find my ability to work with precision to end that cycle. I was able to uncover my core language using Dr. Wolynn's work and connected with a resolution.

I quickly decided I was not going to be one to take out my warrior attitude and go to war with cancer. When examining the relationship here I understood on a visceral level I could not be at odds with parts of myself AND heal from cancer. I practiced presence with myself and extended trust to my own ability to find a solution, I claimed my intuition as an ally. No matter how I felt about it, cancer was here and part of my body, and I had to figure out a way through it, with it, and not against it.

I wanted to be a peacemaker.

Shane Claiborne summarizes what I was feeling beautifully in this quote from The book of Common Prayer "Peacemaking doesn't mean passivity. It is the act of interrupting injustice without mirroring injustice, the act of disarming evil without destroying the evildoer, the act of finding a third way that is neither fight nor flight but the careful, arduous pursuit of reconciliation and justice."

This is exactly how I wanted to stand through this. Interactions with others also came under examination. Jim Rohn famously said that "we are the average of five people we spend the most time with." After examining the data, it's not quite true and goes much deeper and wider extending through social networks up to three degrees of separation.

That's a lot of people! When examining the Framingham Heart Study other insights emerged beyond heart health. It turns out there are studies to show that happiness spreads, depression spreads, obesity spreads.

I clearly see a pattern traveling through large social circles. It explained my internal dialogue about the topic. This isn't about the 5 people I spend the most time with. It's about the vast social network each of us are fortunate to have and I was going to need to rely on my network to help me heal. This seemed overwhelming until I realized it was also empowering.

This means that one family member or family struggle that tends to bring a disproportionate amount of challenges can be balanced with others in your network that can and will be chosen by you. The spotlight was on choosing my friendships and relationships I could lean on while examining my core relationships with family to find out what needed balance. As I moved toward healing and clarity with this I felt empowered. My goal here was to bring both "inner" qualities (qualities of "heart" and intention) and "outer" qualities (how healthcare professionals behave) to my own healing relationship in self-advocacy.

Resiliency was the next core area to address. The first step to this for me was to deal with resistance. I could see how resisting my diagnosis was going to cause more suffering. My stress reduction tool bag was pretty empty at the start, and I was piling on stress without a way to resolve it. As I began to expand my stress reduction with practices like daily prayer, meditation, visualization, deep breathing, purposefully connecting with nature when possible, the fog began to lift, and I could see the work I needed to do more clearly.

Understanding began to emerge when I created space. My own definition of resiliency born out of this experience followed: it is the ability to normalize painful life experiences and realize I am not alone in the pain. Remember that I have been successful in getting through challenges many times before. I realized I have already developed grit through other life experiences. This was an addition to that growth that I can be grateful for. This thought pattern helped me minimize resistance to cancer as a life experience that I could not change.

Acceptance reduces suffering and allows for continued growth and improvement despite the circumstances. This ultimately allowed me to live a purpose driven life in the midst of cancer. I worked thru a book by Laurie Beth Jones (Jones, (1996). *The Path*. Hachette Books). and created my own personal purpose statement.

I found it grounding to have the words written out. Living in alignment with purpose is beautiful at any time, and it is the best set up for bouncing back from difficulties. I found this comes more naturally to me in some aspects of life and less in others. I see great encouragement in the fact that this can be a learned skill in addition to a natural tendency as described in this study of resiliency as a dynamic concept.

Spirituality has been part of my life since childhood in various ways, and I approach spirituality thru a Christian world view. Here I was facing a very different aspect of it: my mortality. Dr. Martinez, my treating acupuncture physician, and a pillar of strength in this journey told me that there are very few people who get to face their mortality early in life and continue living with a different lens to the world. He told me that was unusual and special. I knew right away I could not solve this as an engineering problem, not even as a science problem, from the start I was aware this journey was going to go much deeper than I have ever been spiritually. I have a tendency to over-use my logical brain, and that was about to change.

This was totally different, I wanted to come out on the other end of this journey grateful and humble no matter what happened. It countered logic because the drive to win is natural and strong, yet silent in this process for me. The very first concept I addressed was forgiveness of self and forgiveness of others.

Harboring resentment is poisonous to a person. Dr. Andrew Weil says, "Forgiveness calms the mind and spirit and neutralizes resentment. Resentment fuels one of the most toxic forms of depressive rumination. Running thought loops over and over about past hurts is a major driver of depressive states."

I definitely didn't want to take that with me on this cancer journey. I see forgiveness as a process and not a finite one-time occurrence. I found that being specific regarding a person or an event I needed to forgive was important and sometimes had to be repeated.

I realized I was okay with not getting my old life back and even more, that I was grateful for my new life because I felt myself coming alive and uncovering more of what is vital and sacred to me through this struggle.

Movement has been a constant thread as I raised my kids, regular exercise required some complex scheduling that was not always possible. I started with attending kick boxing classes at the same time as my kids and continued to refine my routine. I found the book by Dr. BJ Fogg (Fogg, BJ (2019) *Tiny Habits, The small changes that change everything*. Boston: Houghton Mifflin Harcourt) helpful in creating a framework for success in being consistent.

The data is clear in suggesting exercise is important for mind, body, emotional and spiritual well-being, it often lowers stress hormones and helps clear thoughts. Movement and exercise is also well researched and substantiated for cancer survivors.

Nutrition is another area where Dr. Fogg's research would be helpful in assisting implementation. I spent a considerable amount of time addressing food for me and my whole family when autism entered our world. One major adjustment I made was going vegan and adding focus to experiencing a meal as an enjoyable practice. I realized the emotional and social aspect was just as important as the nutritional content of a meal. I increased my consumption of fruits and vegetables and added daily juicing.

I never had issues with sleep before, and it became something I watched carefully thru treatment. I realized I was at risk of sleep interruptions due to stress and preemptively used sleep preservation tactics. I did not watch TV before bed and listened to sound recordings at a frequency that promoted sleep. During this time I noticed increased frequency of dreams while being grateful for being able to rest easily in the midst of cancer treatment. Environment was an area I re-evaluated in terms of stress. Our physical environment was already addressed in my treatment of my daughter's autism. During this chapter I focused more on our psychological environment of calm. I rearranged our enclosed patio room to be a healing space without clutter. Comfortable seating and plants indoors as well as a good view of nature from the windows. I purposefully increased my time spent outside and continued with my practices of using green cleaning products in my home.

Future therapies to explore: continue following up with my team of professionals from oncology to acupuncture, integrative medicine and counseling to maintain a healing relationship with myself and my team after treatment.

Remember my long-term goals and tap into traits in addition to intelligence to maintain them. Maintain focus on gratitude and consider adding a gratitude journal. Address movement and exercise as part of daily living without having to depend on routine.

Consider adding herbs for anxiety especially around recurring cancer screening appointments. Possibilities would include: Kava Kava (Piper methysticum), Inositol, Bacopa (Bacopa monnieri), Lemon balm (Melissa officinalis), Passion flower (Passiflora incarnata), Rhodiola (Rhodiola rosea), and Valerian (Valeriana officinalis) (I Help module on anxiety).

Continue exploring research in nutritional science including medical fasting when necessary.

Outcomes: I have experienced the effectiveness of the integrative approach combined with conventional treatment of cancer. I see the emotional aspect often unaddressed along with core areas of health. There have been major realizations and growth along the way.

I would like to illustrate with this air travel story. Did you know that there are rules about when pilots are not allowed to use autopilot while flying an airplane? When an airplane hits turbulence above a very mild level the pilot must take control of the plane. The trouble with autopilot is if it tries to fly the plane on the straight and narrow through significant turbulence, the frequency and magnitude of mindless auto correction would cause structural damage to the aircraft. Sounds dangerous. A pilot, like a patient on the other hand, has the discernment and context to allow the plane to drop within the safety of his knowledge, situational awareness, and experience. A large drop in turbulent air with a softer recovery gives the passengers a smoother ride in addition to avoiding structural damage.

Of course, my mind goes straight to life application. How often we live on autopilot, picking our own "straight and narrow." When turbulence comes, we attempt to hold that line, over correct no matter the cost, and end up with

structural damage to our lives as a result.

Who is piloting us through cancer? How many of us could use the analogy that sometimes a pilot has to allow for a significant fall in order to recover smoothly.

Letting this sink in already gave me a bit of a smoother ride as a bonus.

The Good, The Bad, The Ugly

You literally take your life into your hands with standard of care oncology, but at least all the MDs have licensing boards standing behind them.

Integrative care is definitely a *caveat emptor* proposition too. It includes licensed physicians and naturopaths. It also includes psychologists, masters level mental health practitioners, acupuncturists, energy workers, nutritionists, herbalists, body workers, and a host of others. Some have licenses to practice. Others lack formal credentials.

So long as I brought up credentials, you can verify licenses online. Go to the state licensing board for whatever specialty the provider you're considering claims they have. Make sure they're for real. Check complaints against their license.

The bar is low. Distressingly low, but at least you'll find out if Dr. X got themselves into trouble. There's usually a quick and dirty description of what they did with the caveat that Dr. X doesn't acknowledge fault.

The other thing you'll discover is if the practitioner is misrepresenting themselves. There's one gal who pretends to be a naturopath. Upon closer examination, she isn't. That's unethical at best and fraud at worst.

Most people don't bother to check—or don't know how. The key words are "license verification." If someone is on the up and up, you'll be able to find them listed in the state in which they practice.

This is not necessarily true of energy workers. There are some incredible, magical people out there. Sorting the wheat from the chaff requires diligence.

Back to integrative care clinics. Many of them are out of the country. Oversight varies widely. Some are awesome. Others are just plain crooked.

You really have to do your own research. And you have to find people—hopefully more than one—who actually went to where you're planning on going. This is tougher than it might appear on the surface given patient confidentiality.

Still, it's not impossible.

I joined several integrative care cancer groups on Facebook and spent time reading their files sections and trolling for information. The clinic where I ended up in Reno was the third integrative care venue I'd explored.

Dr. Devlin came highly recommended from more than a single source.

One well-known place in Southern California was sketchy and sleazy. It was pretty clear they were after my money.

You can spend a lot on cancer care. Hundreds of thousands of dollars. Many places prey on the sick and the desperate.

I currently belong to four relevant groups on Facebook:

Healing Cancer Study and Support Group

Breast Cancer Pathways

Always Hope Cancer Protocol Support Group

Fenbendazole Cancer Support Group

These four groups total 112,000 members as of June 2023. Of course, there is overlap. For example, I belong to all four. Still, it's a lot of people. From all over the world. Someone in one of those groups will have gone to the clinic you're considering. Ask for their thoughts and experiences. You'll get far more mileage than reading glowing testimonials on clinic websites.

If possible, visit the venue before obligating yourself.

Be very wary of "package" deals where someone stuffs an entire menu of interventions down your throat with *à la carte* pricing.

That southern California clinic I mentioned earlier tried to do that to me. I had a Zoom meeting with one of their MDs, and delineated which of their interventions I was willing to try. Within seconds of hanging up, I received an email with my "personalized plan." It included a whole lot I'd rejected and bore little resemblance to what I'd talked about with Dr. Shyster.

For example, despite telling them I had my own psychotherapist, someone I had a long history with, they signed me up with their practitioner to the tune of $1200/week. When I looked their person up, turned out she wasn't a licensed psychotherapist at all. Not a psychologist. Not a clinical social worker. Not a marriage, family, child counselor.

Nada.

They also signed me up for hyperbaric oxygen therapy. I live at 8,000 feet. I'd have traveled to roughly sea level to visit their clinic. Hyperbaric O2 therapy could have been dangerous for me given the fact that I live at altitude. Apparently, no one there had any idea about that little ripple.

The experience left me with a very bad taste in my mouth. They hounded me for months afterward. It felt like a used car salesman had my number and was going to keep after me until I "bought or died."

This was before the infusion center fired me, and also before I'd established care with Dr. Devlin.

Be wary of promises.

No one can promise a cure.

Be wary of places that don't highlight a multi-faceted approach that includes exercise, diet, meditation, and other life-affirming practices. There is a scientific basis to integrative care. Ask to see studies highlighting the relevancy of a particular intervention for your type of cancer.

Whether you go the standard of care or integrative route (or a blend), your care provider must be willing to be part of a team that includes you as an active participant.

You get to take part in all decisions.

You can say no.

You can ask for something different.

One of Dr. Devlin's first questions to me was, "What are we doing here?" It's an inclusive question in that he said, "we." It's respectful in that he asked for my input.

He didn't sugarcoat anything, and he did say if I had a recurrence he'd heavy up on suggestions. Honest and forthcoming are good traits in a physician.

A first step for anyone considering integrative treatment is education.

Read books about integrative oncology so you know what it offers. Read more than one. The resource section at the end of this book lists several, any of which would be a solid starting point.

Make sure you can afford to spend several thousand dollars without creating undue stress in your life. There are many ways to raise money. Some people do "Go Fund Me" campaigns. You don't have to go into debt.

A few of the survivor stories stress they spent very little money on their care. So it's not a prerequisite. Diet and exercise are "free," since you have to eat anyway. Choosing healthier food options will cost more, but not that much.

Talk with your family to feel them out about integrative care. If they're going to fight you every step of the way, it's scarcely worth it because of the stress it will produce. Much like sugar, stress feeds cancer.

Many (probably most) people are not in favor of integrative approaches to anything. If an approach hasn't been signed, sealed, and blessed by a traditional MD, it's suspect.

Hell, I started out squarely in the standard of care camp. It didn't last long, but until events began spiraling downhill, it never occurred to me they didn't care about me.

They being my providers.

I'm sure there are some decent oncologists out there, but not as many as you might think. Remember all those social media groups I belong to? Granted, they're mostly the rejects from traditional care and the disgruntled, but there are a whole hell of a lot of us.

It isn't accidental.

Go back to the chapter about cancer as big business and re-read it. We are not "winning" the war on cancer. Far from it. In many ways we're in worse shape than we were fifty years ago.

Before you do anything with either standard of care oncology or integrative oncology, insist on genomic or molecular testing.

You have to have an idea what you're working with, otherwise any treatment isn't much better than a shot in the dark.

I've been told I'm an outlier because the one-two punch of Taxol and Carboplatin wouldn't have had any effect on my tumor. I don't believe it. In addition to integrative care cancer groups, I also belong to one that's specific to my type of uterine cancer. It has a few hundred members since my cancer is relatively rare. Virtually all those women went through standard of care treatment, and the vast majority experienced recurrences pretty early on. Sometimes before they've even finished their initial six chemotherapy treatments.

If Taxol/Carbo had been the proper agent for them, it would have worked far better than that.

Rather than an outlier, I believe I'm actually representative of many women with serous carcinoma.

We need genomic testing FIRST. Before we're poisoned with chemo. Research has already established radiation doesn't alter outcomes for this cancer, so it shouldn't even be a consideration.

Let me close this chapter with a few thoughts.

Just because something is labeled integrative care doesn't make it kosher or good for you.

Just because something is labeled standard of care doesn't make it bad.

No one can do this for you. You have to do your own research, request specific testing, and lobby until someone agrees to do what you know is needed to treat your malignancy.

None of this is easy.

None of it is fair.

We should get to be sick in peace with a bevy of guardian angels watching out for our wellbeing.

It would be lovely, but it isn't realistic.

My PCP has stood in as my guardian angel, and I will be forever grateful for his open-mindedness and compassion. Dr Devlin has as well. My current OB-GYN, too. I'm fortunate to have found three physicians to support me.

This field is evolving quickly. Even the MD who dismissed me from the infusion center reluctantly admitted that a decade from now, chemotherapy won't be part of the arsenal to address cancer. She said it was barbaric, and then she backpedaled furiously.

Sometimes the truth slips out unbidden.

Let's take a look at a survivor story, another interview, and then one more survivor story before we return to my saga.

Noel Watson's Story

Several months before my diagnosis with stage 4, terminal pancreatic cancer on 18th August 2020 I had been aware that my energy levels were reduced for no apparent reason apart from me being in my 70th year. I then began to develop increasing stomach pains which, latterly spread into my back. Initially I thought that this was some sort of gastric problem, so I started taking the usual medications for acid stomach, but these did nothing to alleviate the pain.

However, I found that if I leaned forward then the pain would subside slightly. When the pain had become progressively worse over the ensuing weeks and none of the gastric medications seemed to reduce it, I went to see my GP, who prescribed omeprazole to address the supposed over production of acid plus regular paracetamol for pain control. My doctor also examined me to see whether he could feel any suspicious swelling or inflammation around the stomach area.

He told me he was sure that I had nothing serious to worry about. Very soon after the pain in my stomach and back became so acute that I was rolling around in agony and had to take paracetamol plus ibuprofen constantly every four hours just to get relief for only two hours. It was impossible for me to sleep for more than a couple of hours, and I had to continually reposition myself on the settee in an attempt to reduce the pain.

By this time, I had already started looking up my symptoms online and had deduced pancreatic cancer was a very real possibility. My father had died of pancreatic cancer at the age of 86, and my father-in-law also succumbed to this disease at 82, both of them only living a few months after diagnosis.

My doctor then arranged for me to have an endoscopy in order to diagnose the problem. That evening I had a phone call at about 6.30 pm from a radiographer asking me to arrange an appointment so that he could discuss his findings. I immediately said that I would appreciate it if he could tell me over the phone. He said that they had found a bulky pancreatic tumor, which was consistent with adenocarcinoma. As there was vein and artery involvement, they could not offer me surgery, but chemotherapy might be an option to prolong my life.

In those few seconds my world collapsed around me and devastated my future ambitions. I told him that as my condition was terminal, I did not see the point of prolonging the agony that my cancer would inflict on both me and my family members. I resolved to allow fate to take its course so that I would not be a further burden to my loved ones. I thanked the radiographer for clearly describing my diagnosis and I empathized with him that his job of informing cancer patients must be such a difficult and emotionally challenging task.

My wife gathered our two adult children to our home so that I could tell them the sad and life-changing news we had all dreaded. Fighting back tears I said how very sorry I was to have to tell them I had stage 4, terminal, pancreatic cancer. I told my then 31-year-old son he would now be the new Mr Watson. My 34-year-old daughter sobbed because it was all so unfair.

Several days after this I was contacted by a McMillan nurse who said she would like to come to see whether I was ready to go into hospice or whether my wife would be able to take care of me at home. She was a very kindly lady in her fifties and told me if I went into hospice I would be very well looked after, my pain would be well controlled, and I could enjoy a comfortable stay and even have a bit of fun. I could have as many cream buns as I liked, and patients were able to drink any alcoholic tipple of their choice.

I spoke with the McMillan nurse for a couple of hours and explained I had been a vegetarian for 41 years and was a teetotaler. Most of the time we talked about property and my preoccupation with Bitcoin, so we had an interesting conversation. At the end of her visit, she decided I was not quite ready to go into hospice just yet and she was happy for my wife to look after me until my needs progressed. Fortunately, my wife was well equipped to meet the challenge of looking after me as she had trained as a nurse and been a care home manager for many years looking after the elderly.

My pain had become so unbearable I was prescribed regular doses of Oramorph for which, after a few weeks, I developed a strong loathing. My pain management was then changed to a strong dose of morphine sulphate tablets which enabled me to at least have a few hours' sleep before having to take more tablets.

Little did I know, but my wife had been given my end-of-life morphine syringe driver, which she hid in the top of the wardrobe awaiting its impending usage.

A few weeks after my terminal diagnosis I began to have second thoughts about refusing chemotherapy. I reckoned as I would be dead for a long time, I may as well take advantage of a new experience before my untimely demise. I have always had a somewhat scientific, inquisitive, and logical mind, and I surmised it might be interesting to partake in the chemo experiment.

When I asked my oncologist whether I could start chemotherapy she said I would first need to have a biopsy to determine if the tumor cells were definitely cancerous. This involved having a second endoscopy procedure so that a sample could be taken for analysis.

It was recommended that I did not drive myself to the hospital as I may have some adverse effects from chemotherapy, so my sister-in-law very kindly elected to drive me to and from the hospital some ten miles away. I started my chemo treatment with an infusion of Abraxane followed by Gemcitabine. This process usually took a couple of hours and was repeated three weeks in every four. I actually found that having chemo was quite relaxing, and I took pleasure in knowing nothing was required of me and I had permission to just sit back comfortably and allow the nurses to look after me. After having had a busy working life right up until my illness it felt a real treat to give myself permission to relax and take it easy.

According to my online research I learned I had only a 50% chance of surviving for more than 3 months, which would only take me up to the end of November 2020. It occurred to me that I may never see any spring flowers again, which made me really sad.

Coming to terms with my imminent mortality was such a difficult concept for me to accept, and I became increasingly more depressed. Although I was nearly 70 years old, there were a great many things I still wanted to achieve. Throughout my life I have always gained great pleasure and satisfaction from my personal achievements whether financial or otherwise. The realization I had run out of time to attain even a few more of my goals filled my heart with grief. I reached a mindset where nothing gave me any pleasure. My appetite reduced to practically zero, and I hated the awful tasting Creon enzyme tablets I took to increase my ability to digest the small quantity of food that I did eat. My weight dropped to less than 9 stone.

For the first time in my life my libido became non-existent, yet another aspect of my existence that had been stolen from me by my cancer diagnosis. As my depression became my new normal, I believed I would never ever experience happiness again. I was convinced my misery would only cease with my inevitable and untimely death.

Although it was casually mentioned the morphine sulphate tablets might give me constipation, I was not prepared for the agony that entailed. In desperation, my wife phoned the McMillan nurses asking whether someone could give me an enema to relieve my agonizing condition. As it was Sunday, and no nurses were available, my wife was told I could obtain an enema from my local chemist and that it was quite an easy procedure to follow. The success and relief from suffering achieved by means of the enema was immense.

I have been incredibly fortunate that throughout my cancer journey my wife has always been there to help me in any way she can. She hated seeing me in such a state of despair and suggested it might be possible to raise my mood if I were to ask the doctor to prescribe an anti-depression medicine. After a few weeks of taking citalopram, my depression was significantly repressed and I was more able to mentally accept my condition. I continued taking citalopram for about twelve months, by which time I had regained my will to live and realized that I indeed had some control over my own destiny.

After taking a chemo combination of Gemcitabine and Abraxane for about four months a CT scan showed that my tumor had increased in size from 6 cm to 10.4 cm, which was a great cause of concern. When I walked it felt as though there was a heavy lead weight pulling inside my stomach. My oncologist changed my chemo regime to Gemcitabine and the oral chemo tablet Capecitabine in an attempt to shrink the tumor.

I was curious to learn more about pancreatic cancer and cancer in general to see whether I could do anything to prolong my life. It was at this stage in my research I learned about the case of Joe Tippens, who had incurable small cell lung cancer and who was sent home to die in 2016 with a life expectancy of less than three months.

With nothing left to lose, he embarked on treatment suggested by a veterinary surgeon friend with a repurposed medicine, namely fenbendazole, for deworming and treating cancer in dogs and large animals. After only four months of treatment with a low dose of fenbendazole he had a CT scan which revealed he was totally free from cancer! Before taking fenbendazole, in an earlier scan his body lit up like a Christmas tree!

Joe Tippens was also taking part in a trial to try to extend his life along with 1,100 other cancer patients. At the end of the trial, he was the only one who had responded positively to the trial, and he put it down to the fact that he was the only one who was, without the doctor's knowledge, taking fenbendazole. Joe is still very much alive and thriving seven years later and has been responsible for many thousands of people following his protocol with a multitude of consequent success stories. The Facebook fenbendazole cancer support group now has over 65,000 members.

I was intrigued by Joe Tippen's story and immediately bought some fenbendazole tablets from a recommended online distributor. One month before my next scan I started taking 4 X 500 mg tablets of fenbendazole every day, a dose which I still take now. This combination of the chemo drugs Gemcitabine and Capecitabine and the repurposed dog wormer caused my tumor to shrink from 10.4 cm back down to 6 cm. I continued taking the fenbendazole plus chemo for another three months during which time my tumor had reduced still more to 2.5 cm.

I was overjoyed.

Although my tumor had decreased in size the Capecitabine was giving me severe neuropathy in my feet. When I put my feet on the ground it was as though I was walking on broken glass. My oncologist recommended I cease taking the Capecitabine chemo medicine so my feet could recover. I asked her whether there were other nerve blocker medicines I could take instead of amitriptyline, which didn't seem to work, so she agreed that I could try Gabapentin instead.

I was unhappy about not continuing with Capecitabine as I was afraid my tumor could experience a substantial growth. My oncologist responded by saying if I kept taking Capecitabine, I could suffer additional negative effects from the treatment other than neuropathy.

As I had feared my next scan showed an increased tumor size from 2.5 cm to 3.5 cm, which was not the result for which I was hoping. I told my oncologist I would like to try alternative medicines to maintain or reduce the tumor size. I asked her whether she could monitor any medicines I added to my protocol to ensure there were no contraindications.

She said she couldn't give me any help or advice regarding alternative medicines as she had no knowledge of them herself! I mentioned to her that conventional chemotherapy only treated the main body of the tumor but not the stem cells which could not even be detected by a CT scan, so I thought I should seek medicines that were able to kill off these stem cells.

She said that cancer was not a simple disease and that it was always going to be difficult to treat!

She expressed no desire whatsoever to encourage me to research alternative therapies which may well extend my life or alleviate my condition. No advice or encouragement of any sort were offered.

She said she would arrange a blood test for me and book me in for another scan in a few months' time after which she would decide on any further treatment.

Although I am very grateful for our NHS, I'm disappointed and frustrated our doctors and oncologists rely only on conventional medicine with complete lack of knowledge and disregard of any complementary alternatives.

It is my opinion many more lives could be saved by people taking control of their own destiny by seeking the vast number of alternative medicines that can be sourced and purchased from online stores. It is a sad fact that the majority of people put their trust in the conventional medicine machine and totally overlook the fact that they can and are capable of increasing their chances of survival by seeking alternative medicines.

I heard about my next supplementary medicine from one of my wife's friends who is a dedicated exponent of chlorine dioxide which he has been using himself for the last 20 years. Its popularity was gained by Jim Humble who used it to cure several people of malaria in a matter of only a few hours and then found out it could cure many other ailments as well. Chlorine dioxide solution has been called the universal antidote by NASA, as it is capable of curing or alleviating literally hundreds of different diseases and conditions.

I watched a few Andreas Kalcker videos on chlorine dioxide solution and browsed through his free e-books and was immediately blown away by all the information within.

I eagerly started the Andreas Kalcker protocol for cancer which is 7 mls of chlorine dioxide taken with half a cup of water 7 times per day. I started on a lower dose over the first day to ensure that I didn't suffer from the Herx Heimer effect of possible sickness or upset stomach my friend told me about. I rapidly increased my dose to the full 50 mls per day, and I suffered no ill effects from taking this relatively high dose.

Throughout my illness I have tried to stage my physical strength in order to ascertain whether any particular medication was having a beneficial effect on me. Before my illness, I was easily able to do 10 press ups, but 20 months after my diagnosis I was totally unable to do even one single press up, so I used this as a benchmark for any further improvement.

After only four days of taking chlorine dioxide, I tested myself by trying press ups and to my delight I found that I could do one press up easily! Three weeks after taking daily chlorine dioxide solution I found that I could do 10 press ups which was an unbelievable improvement.

Before my illness, I always used to run small distances everywhere. Since my diagnosis, although I was able to walk, whenever I tried to run my legs felt like lead weights, as though they didn't belong to me. After just one week of taking chlorine dioxide, I was now able to run around the garden even quite quickly and my legs actually began to feel progressively normal and as though I owned them once more.

Truly remarkable progress, and I resolved to carry on the protocol permanently.

I had been taking about 50 mls per day of chlorine dioxide solution plus Gemcitabine infusions and fenbendazole before my next CT scan. I was relieved and delighted to hear that this scan showed that my pancreatic tumor had reduced from 3.5 cm down to 2.7 cm. This was brilliant news for me as my previous scan had shown an increase in size from 2.5 cm up to 3.5 cm. To have reversed the process and actually reduced the tumor size once more was a real game changer.

It would seem to me that the addition of the chlorine dioxide solution (CDS) four weeks before this scan was the essential ingredient that was responsible for not only stopping the growth of my tumor but also reversing the process.

My next new discovery and vitally important alternative treatment was dimethyl sulfoxide (DMSO). DMSO alleviates or cures an astonishing 300 diseases or ailments and is also beneficial in healing many types of cancer. I was absolutely delighted so far with my very fortuitous progress regarding my battle with pancreatic cancer. I felt much more in control of my own destiny and am truly grateful alternative treatment came to my rescue in my moment of need.

Over the ensuing months I continued my online research regarding all types of cancer. I watched a multitude of videos, read copious articles on PubMed and joined over 30 Facebook cancer groups in order to extend my knowledge of cancer. I researched and trialled many well tolerated, affordable natural products and repurposed medicines, which I added to my growing cancer beating protocol. I used PubMed as my bible as it contains copious amounts of information gathered from peer reviewed scientific papers.

My most recent CT scan followed a chemo break of 3 1/2 months, so I was eager to know whether my supplements alone could maintain a stable tumor size. I was profoundly relieved to learn my tumor had remained stable with no metastases.

This is a clear indication to me my supplements have now taken over the role of stopping further tumor progression in its tracks without the assistance of chemotherapy. It could have been that the chemotherapy had stopped working many months ago and that my supplements alone would have produced the same results; I have no way of telling.

Based on these results my oncologist was quite happy for me to continue another three months chemo break before my next scan. She did however mention that although my tumor had not increased in size this time, I should not expect any further reduction and that my cancer was still terminal!

34 months after my stage 4 pancreatic cancer diagnosis I am not only surviving but am thriving and immensely grateful I am still alive. Without the influence of chemotherapy, I am

now stronger than I have been for more than three years. At the age of nearly 73 I resumed working on my property portfolio, which involves quite heavy building work, plumbing, carpentry, plastering and a great deal of painting.

Here is my present supplement protocol. The dosage is one tablet per day unless otherwise stated.

I take 2,000 mg of fenbendazole per day (4 X 500 mg tablets),

45 mls of chlorine dioxide solution (CDS) (5 X 9 mls) per day each dose mixed with 1 ml of DMSO diluted in half a cup of soya milk or water.

About 16 grams of taurine also diluted with fruit juice per day (2 X 8 grams).

Vitamins

A 10,000 IU

B12 1,000 mcg

D 4,000 IU

E 400 IU soft gels

K 2,600 mcg

Turmeric X 2 tablets per day (each tablet contains 1,260 mg turmeric, organic ginger 100 mg, organic black pepper 20 mg).

high strength melatonin 60 mg every night and 60 mg in the morning

turkey tail mushroom 10,000 mg

berberine 1,000 mg

milk thistle (for liver protection) 2,000 mg

tudca 500 mg

omega 3 800 mg

alpha lipoic acid 500 mg

magnesium 100 mg

Ivermectin 12 mg per day

serrapeptase 2 X 120,000 SPU tablets per day.

IP-6 inositol hexaphosphate 60 mg

I also drink green tea and ginger tea as they are both known to kill cancer stem cells which is the Holy Grail of any cancer treatment but not addressed by chemotherapy, radiotherapy, or surgery.

I tell as many people as I can about the beneficial healing effects of these complementary products that I believe have been responsible for my own good fortune. I have become a keyboard warrior posting content on a multitude of Facebook cancer groups regarding my unusual longevity surviving stage 4 pancreatic cancer in the hope I can encourage fellow sufferers that they too may benefit from an integrative approach to cancer.

I now look upon my cancer diagnosis as a privilege and even a blessing!

My reasoning for this is that before I became ill, I had neither the knowledge, experience, or motivation to help other people with their various illnesses or afflictions.

I believe the most important thing we can accomplish during our time on earth is to help other people or even better to be instrumental in saving their lives.

As I have now gained credibility regarding my own personal journey with cancer, I can share my newly gained knowledge and experience with other cancer patients with the hope that they too may have the opportunity of experiencing my good fortune.

Real Hope for Cancer Patients

Regarding pancreatic cancer my oncologist left me in no doubt whatsoever that my stage 4 pancreatic cancer is terminal and all she can do is to extend my life as long as possible by chemotherapy. When the chemo stops working, which she tells me it inevitably will, I will have to accept my demise. This is the default prognosis given by our NHS oncologists to anyone suffering from stage 4 inoperable pancreatic cancer.

Even when one has the benefit of surgery statistically pancreatic cancer can often return 12 months after the operation. This is the prognosis according to the standard of care (SOC) treatment given by our oncologists. This presents the cancer patient with little or no hope of any long-term survival. If the patient accepts their oncologist is correct, then they know they are on borrowed time until their cancer inevitably defeats them.

My belief however, after discovering supplements, is patients can take control over their cancer and be responsible for their own destiny. Without immediate and direct action by the patient their brief window of hope diminishes by the days or weeks ahead. With a 50% mortality rate in the first 3 months of a stage 4 pancreatic cancer diagnosis, we do not have the luxury of time to just wait and see what happens.

It breaks my heart every time I hear of patients or their caregivers, who have been slow to act and then found it was too late to take control of their own destiny by means of alternative medicine. Deciding to try a few supplements when one is in hospice and given only a few weeks to live is not the best time to realize one should have acted sooner. If people come across my posts fresh from diagnosis, they may realize there is indeed very realistic hope they can take control of their own lives and enjoy a better outcome. This may spur them into action to immediately commence the addition of supplementary medicines to their existing chemo regime.

Using supplementary medicine in addition to chemotherapy, we can reduce the tumor size and possibly prevent metastases. For longer term healing we need to kill the cancer stem cells by supplements and nutrition as neither chemo nor radiation can do this.

We can survive for many years living with a stable tumor which is unable to metastasize. To achieve their best outcome, we need to encourage pancreatic cancer patients to act immediately and proactively to extend their life as long as possible.

The standard of care in our hospitals is woefully limited to chemo, radiation, and surgery due to the monopoly and stranglehold of Big Pharma, which has blighted our medical treatment for over a hundred years. Our oncologists are prevented from prescribing any medicine that has not been approved by virtue of a clinical trial as their insurance would not cover them for any harmful effects of these medicines. There is no financial motivation for the pharmaceutical companies to spend millions of dollars on clinical trials unless they could profit from the patent. There is no money to be made from off patent, repurposed, or natural products that would jeopardize Big Pharma's trillion-dollar industry.

My 'impossible' dream is that whenever a cancer patient is given their diagnosis, they are also told in writing something like, 'We will give you the best medical attention available to us within the constraints and permissions of the pharmaceutical industry. However, it may be in your interests to consider the addition of some well-chosen supplementary medicines to your treatment plan. It is considered that an integrative medical approach has often been found to yield the best possible outcome.'

Our paramount agenda surely must be that of staying alive in the long run, and as we heal our quality-of-life improves too. At the age of nearly 73 I now spend much of my free time spreading the word of supplementary medicine to thousands of cancer sufferers on dozens of Facebook cancer groups.

I do this not for any financial gain but out of sheer gratitude I am still not only surviving but thriving. I am just so very grateful for my accidental and fortuitous discovery of the wonderful healing attributes of supplementary medicines.

There are a great number of links to videos and information on alternative medicine on my Facebook home page and I am always grateful to hear from anyone who I may have the privilege of helping.

Here is the sequel to one of my Facebook cancer group posts ten months ago following my exposition of the monopoly of Big Pharma which is endemic within the trillion-dollar cancer industry.

It looks as though I may be making waves within the cancer community, because I received literally thousands of notifications after that post. This gives me the strength and resolution to redouble my efforts in bringing awareness to the whole cancer community of the remarkable positive healing attributes of alternative medicines that are sadly given zero recognition by the medical industry.

Although I am very grateful for our NHS, I'm disappointed and frustrated that our doctors and oncologists rely only on conventional medicine with a complete lack of knowledge and disregard for any complementary alternatives.

It is my opinion many more lives could be saved by people taking control of their own destiny by seeking the vast number of alternative medicines that can be sourced and purchased from online stores. It is a sad fact that the majority of people put their trust in the conventional medicine machine and totally overlook the fact that they can and are capable of increasing their chances of survival by seeking alternative medicines.

Note from Ann: Noel has his own FB page. He'd love it if you joined.

Mark Sean Taylor Interview

Mark Sean Taylor runs the Patient Led Oncology Trials group on FB. He graciously agreed to an interview for this book.

Mark has spent 20 years working in finance and technology, working in London, New York, Hong Kong, Istanbul and Sao Paulo. Diagnosed with minimal residual disease pancreatic cancer through circulating tumour cells in 2016, he was rejected for standard of care medicine, as the level of cancer was below what mainstream medicine recognizes for a formal diagnosis. He has since spent more than $500,000 USD on treatments and tests at some of the top medical institutions around the world, learning the approaches of some of the world's leading integrative doctors. He is an avid cancer researcher, experimenting with a broad range of modalities from personalised cancer vaccines through to various energy healing modalities in Central America, to the use of psychedelics for trauma healing. He now works with and advises some of the top integrative cancer clinics over the world and is currently being trained in the use of *psychedelics for compassionate inquiry under the guidance of Gabor Mate. He blogs about his findings through:*

https://www.facebook.com/groups/patientledoncologytrials

Interview

Mark: What's the concept of the book you're writing?

Ann: To say I had a miserable time with the American oncology system would be a gross understatement. No one should have to live through what I did. If I have an overarching zeitgeist for *Alive*, it's to encourage people to stand up for themselves and ask questions.

Mark: Yes, totally.

Ann: There's so much you can do to help yourself. I belong to a number of online cancer groups. In some specific to my type of cancer, there's a trend to take what the oncologist says as gospel and to become more a passive recipient than an active partner in your care.

I have no idea if this book will find an audience, but I hope it does.

Mark: I'll read it.

Ann: Thank you. Let's segue into these questions. You have a background in international finance and technology. How did you become interested in integrative cancer care?

Mark: I had a difficult period with work and working on an MBA. Flying between Hong Kong and Istanbul, I had a burnout, breakdown. The symptoms didn't disappear. I was experiencing stomach pains. When I explored this further, they found lesions in my pancreas and circulating tumor cells considered to be suspected pancreatic cancer from the genetic analysis. It was very early, too early to be treated by an oncologist. Thankfully, it meant I had to delve into ways to heal myself with integrative medicine. At the start, I didn't totally trust it. I was surprised how much information was out there. And then I went on to collect data from other patients, which is sort of what I do now.

Ann: When were you diagnosed with circulating tumor cells? 2015?

Mark: 2016

Ann: So it's been almost a decade. Do you have evidence there's any cancer left in your system?

Mark: My chemo markers are lower than they have been. Circulating tumor cells are low as well.

Ann: Which test are you using?

Mark: RGCC and recently I visited a clinic in Romania that has its own machine.

Ann: So not one I'd be familiar with. Not Signatera or Guardant.

Mark: Those aren't particularly good for early stage disease from my experience

Ann: You could say the things you've done for yourself have been a success.

Mark: Yes, my markers are quite low. It took me six years of traveling the world. I've had a lot of treatment, perhaps more than anyone. In some ways I view myself as a lab rat. It was only until last year when I got my body into a state where the markers could fall naturally.

Ann: For me, it's been a mindset thing. Maybe it's silly, perhaps an ostrich approach, but the mind-body connection is powerful.

Mark: Yes. It's being proven now. I went on a mission to understand the results of these newer studies. Some integrative oncologists have stepped outside of standard of care to pioneer other methods to make things work. I spent a lot of money with them. In the interest of not bankrupting myself, I began studying about natural methods to allow the body to heal.

Heart rate variability can be tracked. Studies show it correlates with cancer outcomes. What you sometimes see with cancer patients is they're never able to reduce that variability. Their bodies are in a constant state of fight or flight.

Using the body and mind collectively to heal is key.

Ann: This is one of the points I make in the book, that chronic stress is not your friend. A constant glucocorticoid cascade keeps people in an aroused state. It basically just feeds cancer.

Mark: Yes. You can carry on treatment in that state, but the interventions aren't fun and they're expensive. Now that we have the technology to monitor heart rate, hopefully it will see greater use. What was historically an anomaly (why them and not me), is becoming mainstream. The data now shows you're not doing that well because of a measurable item, that can be tracked on your Apple watch or aura ring.

I had to change careers, relationships, places to live, friendship groups in order to remove some of the stresses of life. This is becoming more accepted, and people would be well served to get themselves into a state where they can actually heal. Kelly Turner's *Radical Remission* discusses this at length.

Soon we'll have greater and greater numbers of people who find ways to heal themselves.

Ann: Long before Radical Remission, there was a book titled, *Love, Medicine, and Miracles* by Bernie Siegel MD. It was revolutionary at the time because Dr. Siegel, an oncologist, was advising patients to be active partners in their care, to exercise, to meditate. He put together probably the first—maybe the only—support group led by an oncologist.

Mark: I'll have a look at it. This is becoming mainstream. Staff at the high-end integrative cancer clinics are espousing whole person care with meditation, exercise, and so on.

Ann: Not where I was, but then I only found integrative care after traditional care booted me. Do you believe there's a place for Standard of Care oncology? If so, where does it fit into treatment?

Mark: A very good question. Something I think about a lot. If you flip the question and are running a national health service or an insurance company, there has to be some management of costs and procedures. Countries need to manage budgets, and you need some level of standards.

Ann: We don't have that problem in the U.S., but keep going. Our health system is for profit all the way. Insurance companies rake in double digit profits every single year.

Mark: Amazing. There is a need. When you're rolling out chemo and immunotherapies, they're complex drugs. From a drugmaker's point of view you need some standards. I get that side of it. Is the balance too far? In the controls around standard of care. In the past medical knowledge doubled every 50 years. Today, it doubles every few months. The difference between standard of care and experimental doctors will continue to widen, because of this fact. In three to five years, you can almost guarantee being kept alive—not necessarily a cure—by various interventions.

It's a bit like HIV where they found ways to keep patients alive. There had to be a level of activism to turn the protease inhibitors into standard of care. We're not far off that point in cancer.

Ann: There was an article in the NYT about a month ago written by a young breast cancer survivor. She made the point that today we have the technology to move from one intervention to another, hopscotching to keep people alive. She also made the point that these interventions are only available to a select few.

Mark: True. There are countries like India and places in Africa where some people receive no medication because the drugs are so expensive. So unfortunately treatments are likely to differ for those that have money and those that don't. But we can still work to improve outcomes at the same price point.

Ann: They really don't need to be that expensive. Look at the difference between drug prices in Canada and the U.S. What advice would you give someone newly diagnosed with cancer?

Mark: Very good question. Go online and find groups like my Patient Led Oncology Trials or Healing Cancer Study and support group or Jane McLelland's group. Meet other patients. Get yourself educated. Work on the mind-body side. If you're stage one, no need to panic. If you're stage four, you have some difficult decisions to make regarding how much you want to spend on integrative care—if you decide to go that route.

Ann: A number of people have been given terminal diagnoses and they're still alive and kicking thanks to integrative care.

Mark: Yes. Exactly.

Ann: Would you advise someone to educate themselves before their follow-up meeting with an oncologist?

Mark: It's difficult. Time is an issue. If you have stage four pancreatic cancer, you might have seven months to live. They're going to rush you into chemo. To get yourself educated enough in even seven months is difficult. So, how you get up to speed and how you have confidence in talking with an oncologist isn't that easy. You have to take a little bit of a leap of faith. If you have a stage one melanoma, you have a lot more latitude. If it's a terminal case, and the person is going straight into high dose chemo, you really want to take a step back and strategize. Look at clinical trials. See what you can afford to spend on experimental treatments. Do that up front before you go the chemo route because once you go the chemo route it will destroy your body and the path to healing becomes far more difficult.

Ann: That's all true. I've come across many practitioners who say patients who come to them clean have a far more robust response to integrative treatments.

Mark: I work in clinics now. Nearly 100% of the patients who come to us are damaged from cancer treatments. Hemoglobin problems, white blood cell problems, damaged kidneys, neuropathies. I think that needs to be talked about more. Chemo has pretty horrific side effects. It truly does damage you. It's a rare person who emerges unscathed. There are ways to limit the side effects, but it needs a fundamental charge to move away from maximum tolerable doses, when lower doses will effect positive change too with far fewer side effects.

Ann: Would you advise people to request genomic or molecular testing prior to treatment?

Mark: Certainly. Genomics testing should be standard of care. Get whatever you can free. Not everyone will come up with a mutation you can target. With private testing, you can do so much more. NextGen Oncology, BostoneGene, DATAR, RGGC all provide information that can help your outcomes. They yield so much more information regarding what your tumor would respond to.

Ann: What is a good working definition of integrative oncology?

Mark: To me, it's anything above and including standard of care. Integrative might not be the best word. Not sure there's a right word to describe it. Anything with evidence behind it to help you on your journey.

Ann: So, more of a whole person approach?

Mark: Yes. Could be meditation, could be exercise. Could be supplements, could be cancer vaccines. Could be testing. But not excluding standard of care. So it could be someone doing IVC with standard of care.

Ann: Describe how you view the mind-body connection as it relates to the development of cancer and other diseases.

Mark: This is something I've started researching more and more. There's a definite link between trauma and cancer. When I talk with patients, I often see a divorce, a death in the family, a breakdown in work. Other causes can be toxins, alcohol, cigarettes, bacteria, viruses, fungi. A whole host of things can contribute to the development of a cancering process. The body is basically overwhelmed and is going through the process of developing cancer. We know now there's a clear link between heart rate variability to measure whether you're in an activated state or healing. To me, it's getting your body into a healing state for long enough so it can heal.

I've seen evidence that a specific trauma can cause tumor growth in a particular organ. If you think it through, it's what Chinese medicine talks about with emotion being tied to various organs. People with autoimmune disorders will tell you they can feel trauma in specific places in their bodies. Some psychedelics, like psilocybin and MDMA, are good for treating trauma. EMDR too.

Cancer patients should do work to release suppressed traumas in their body as part of the healing process.

I've done trauma healing myself, and I've noticed the same concept happening in my body. It's like a power center that forms around the trauma.

Ann: It's protected, like a shell.

Mark: Exactly. This has been denied by the conventional world forever, but now the world has become more accepting. The way to heal from trauma is you have to relive it by going into the bodily sensation. It must be felt where it's lodged. This relates to the concept of chi as we direct it to a particular bodily location to heal. Trauma is a dissociation where the pain of that memory is too strong, and you disconnect from the body. Healing is only possible once you're in a safe space and can go back into that trauma, experience it, and let it go.

Ann: That's the healing methodology for PTSD and for phobias. It's a structured exposure.

Mark: Yes, similar concept. It's also a meditation technique, gradually entering the uncomfortable zone and staying with it until the sensation dissipates. It also acknowledges traumas can pass through generations, so going back through the family history of trauma is also useful.

Ann: Do you see value in mapping the matriarchal and patriarchal lines in a modified trance so you can figure out what happened when and go in and try to heal it.

Mark: That's the method my therapist used with me. It works very well. There is a physical connection between the brain and the body. If the trauma is severe enough, you're not going into that part of the brain at all, which short circuits connections between that part of the brain and the body.

Ann: For what it's worth, I believe people were more in tune with their bodies fifty or sixty years ago before there was all this screen time.

Mark: Yes, it's a distraction process. It's a dissociation from the body. We need to be better anchored in our bodies. More self-aware.

Ann: One of your current projects involves the use of psychedelics in managing mood. Please describe what you're doing and how you envision it helping cancer patients.

Mark: It started with me using them to get myself back on track. I'd lost the ability to focus on anything, and to me they were immensely healing. I went from a place of total dysfunction to feeling better than I had for years. The studies coming from NYU and Johns Hopkins are very powerful. They support an 80% reduction in anxiety and depression. If you look at Kelly Turner's findings, releasing suppressed emotions is a benefit as is a spiritual connection. Increasing positive emotion is another benefit. It can even improve heart rate variability. We talk about mindset being so important. This is the one thing strong enough to impact terminal cancer patients' moods. Many other methods are not quick enough or powerful enough. Between the shock of the diagnosis and the horrifically difficult treatments, there's no space to get better emotionally. Talk therapy won't work fast enough. Antidepressants are a band aid.

Ann: Are we talking micro-dose psilocybin? Or ketamine here?

Mark: No. Full dose psilocybin. The mechanism isn't fully understood. You need a trained facilitator. Their role is much like a mother caring for a child. To support them and allow them to work through trauma, you need to relive and re-experience the trauma in the body. This is not an easy place for many people to hold, and I certainly don't recommend doing it alone. There's a complicated discussion how this will be integrated into standard of care. It might be rolled out as soon as 2025, but four or five hours with a therapist is expensive. Not sure how they'll manage that.

Civilizations from thousands of years ago were doing things like this as part of their daily life. They still are with tribes in the Amazon and places like that.

Ann: Let's talk about rituals. I'm not sure how it is where you live, but rituals have all but fallen by the wayside. A few things still happen here, but nothing like there used to be. I believe rituals were what bonded us together as families and as friends.

Mark: Yes, Gabor Mate has just written a book, *The Body Keeps the Score*, and he talks about the world we live in as being quite toxic. We've lost a sense of connection. We've all moved into cities. No traditions that bind us. I do see a movement happening to bring that back. Yoga and meditation are examples of group endeavors. How to bring meaning back into our lives.

One thing people need to understand is no matter where they get standard of care treatment, they won't get a think-outside-the-box type of MD like Dr. House. They'll get a very similar treatment from Mayo as they'll get from a much smaller, less famous clinic.

Ann: This has been productive. Is there anything else you'd like readers to know?

Mark: I think we covered most of it. Thank you.

Amanda's Story

Loving who you are, where you are, is the key to living your best life. That sounds overly simple, but it is the foundation for healing and building a life that expresses your uniqueness. A life that is designed by you, for you. Living your best life means something different for each one of us. It is open to interpretation, and has no boundaries.

I used to think life would be easier if it came with a personalized guide on how to survive whatever was encountered on your path. One profound day, at my absolute rock bottom, I realized that I was missing the point. Life is yours to create as you choose. There are no rules, only unlimited choices. Nothing more, nothing less, I was entirely responsible for the life I had created. At that moment, I realized I had the power to change course, and chart a new direction.

Life is actually incredibly simple, but we tend to complicate it through fear. We are conditioned to stay safe, rather than live out loud. We are influenced by our parents, our culture and society to fit in, to not rock the boat and to do what we're told. Many of us live unconsciously, comfortably going through the motions of a familiar life which was designed by someone else.

Everything from the clothes we wear to the foods we eat to the way we decorate our homes, are in some way influenced by someone else.

I tend to use the path or journey analogy to describe the adventure of a life on this planet. I use myself as the example, not because I'm special, but because I have a unique understanding of how I arrived here, typing these words, in the 97th version of this chapter. The inner critic is quietly working in the background, while the perfectionist struggles to get it "right."

Transitioning into the heroine of my story didn't happen overnight, but shutting the door on victim mode was sudden and final. I was exhausted from fighting and holding it together for everyone else, while suffering in silence.

I found myself in a prison that I had created, but I was standing at the door of my prison cell, realizing it had been open the whole time. I had stage 4 breast cancer. I was dying but I wasn't finished with this life. There is nothing quite like facing your mortality and realizing you don't want your story to end just yet.

Physically, I was feeling fantastic. My hair was growing back. Everyone thought I was through the worst part of treatment. I no longer received the pity stares or the knowing looks from those who had been there. I was having an identity crisis. Who was I now that chemo and surgery were over? The perception was I had done amazingly; that I was a warrior; that I had kicked cancer's ass. Mentally, the struggle was raging. I felt like a fraud and that when I died, I was going to have let everyone down. It seemed to me, I was well on my way to be a first class loser.

That day was my breaking point, the day I finally let go and began to trust. I was lying under a tree, in a full blown breakdown, sobbing hysterically, wondering what it would be like as I began to die. I was alone and struggling with intrusive thoughts I couldn't stop. I asked for help, and it wasn't long before I heard in my own voice: Do you want to live?

It was one of those life altering experiences people talk about. A moment when everything suddenly makes sense. I realized that my desire to live was just a little stronger than the pull to give up. I had made the decision to step forward and steer my ship. I had no idea what was going to happen, but I knew I wanted to live the best life possible, for the remainder of the time I had.

The unconscious way most of us live is shaped by the teachings and beliefs of those we trusted or who we looked up to. Our own experiences add another layer and help build the box of beliefs that shapes who we are and how we fit into the world. We learn to cope. We learn how to keep ourselves comfortable, and life moves along a fairly predictable path. Until it doesn't, and everything we know is tossed aside. That day, I dropped all of the baggage, dumped out the contents, and took a good look back to understand how the hell I managed to guide myself here.

When I was eight, my sister was born, and my papa got sick. It was the first time my world was absolutely shattered. It was then I realized that people come and go, and that your heart can be broken. I experienced grief, and the fear of being abandoned took root.

I was old enough to learn about the heartaches those I loved had lived through. I saw the world outside of my limited view as a place of sorrow, pain, and trauma. I began to see that not everyone grew up with love. I saw the dark side of humanity as the veil had been lifted on the idyllic life of my childhood. I realized I was different from other kids. I didn't know my biological father. I heard the word illegitimate used to describe me, and while I didn't understand, I recognized that it wasn't a compliment.

I was fortunate to live on a farm, but it left me isolated from a social group. Chores and responsibilities were expected and if not completed, there was no opportunity for downtime. If I didn't work hard enough, or do a good job, I was punished. I feared being rejected and feared not being liked. I feared being abandoned and felt I was the problem. Being raised to be compliant and agreeable set up a pattern to be that way with everyone. A people pleaser is not born, we are made.

As I matured, I began to understand why my family was the way they were. My grandfather died suddenly when my mom was 5, my nana was a young widow. My aunts experienced severe abuse at the hands of their husbands, and my mom was left a single mother by a selfish, broken man.

I began to recognize the strength, resilience, and fortitude it takes to make the best life possible under dire circumstances. I took some of those qualities, tucked them away, and set out to live a quiet life, free from drama, struggle, and heartache. Fear was the driving force behind playing small, staying close to home, and hiding behind accepted social norms. Fear is a very shaky foundation to build a life on.

With my default settings, I set out on the familiar road I saw everyone else travel. By the time I was 24, I was married with 2 children, we had bought our first home, and on the outside, everything was as it should be. The truth was we were emotionally stunted humans, fumbling around trying to make a go of marriage. When you come from a long line of people who made the best of their circumstances, failure is not an option. The problem was we didn't know what to do. I was suffering, my husband was suffering, but we kept going, miserable and without any real idea how to make anything better.

Looking back, we did the best we knew how with the tools we had. There is no way to move beyond what you know unless a way presents itself. I'm not going to go into detail about what happened, but a challenge came along which forced us to move forward. All of the wounds, the hidden insecurities and fears I had tucked away, spilled out as the foundation of our marriage collapsed.

Instead of picking up the pieces and rebuilding, I sat in the rubble and played the victim. It was a comfortable role that was far easier than taking responsibility for the part I played in the collapse. Being the victim gave me an opportunity to be supported and to be the heroine. It was an opportunity for me to express how hurt I was by the men in my life by pointing the finger squarely at my husband.

For weeks, the anger that consumed me, held us hostage. I couldn't let go. I couldn't see a way out of the box I trapped us in. Something had to give in order to move beyond the misery. In a defining moment, my husband, who was finally tired enough of my garbage, asked me what I needed to happen to move forward. No one had asked me that question. No one had taken the time to ask me what I wanted. All I knew was I wanted to stop feeling angry and to move forward. I didn't know how.

I truly believe that at this moment in time, my cancer was given the perfect ingredients to begin to grow.

There was relief in deciding to reach out to a marriage counselor. I packed up all of my emotional belongings, preparing to work on the marriage. My goal was to move out of the sadness and rage that had taken over my life. I wanted help but had no idea what to do to move towards happiness. I also wanted to be validated that I was worthy and that I was justified in being so angry. It didn't go that way.

After asking us both about the type of family we grew up in, the counselor zeroed in on my childhood. She had the audacity to ask me how I felt about not knowing my biological father, and how I felt about losing my papa. She asked about my relationship with myself. I felt attacked, vulnerable, and that she placed all of the blame squarely on me.

I left with a new conviction to figure this out myself. It didn't dawn on me until years later, while reflecting back, that she actually gave me a key - I was responsible for me. I didn't want to revisit the past. I wanted to move forward, to learn how to feel better, to move out of sadness. I needed space to figure out where I was heading.

I set out to learn everything I could about people and what made them tick. I saw the brokenness, the sadness, the hurt in others. My world expanded beyond my limited view. I started to understand that hurt people hurt other people. I was changing. Life was getting better. I understood that as I changed, the world around me would begin to reflect that change. I took psychology courses, learned hypnosis, and EFT Tapping. I was my experiment, everything I learned was being tested out on myself. It was exhilarating and I was going to change the world.

For a few years, I moved through the motions of raising my children, working at a job I thought was perfect, all the while thinking I was living the life. Inner work is deep, and I had only scratched the surface. I'd reached a plateau.

I regressed back into the old me, the victim stuck in the prison I created, with no pressing need to move on. I was comfortable in the stuckness. It was familiar and required no effort. I hated it, but I didn't know what was next. It was easier to stay, than to reinvent myself. I was being squeezed, but the pressure wasn't great enough to cause me to move.

The universe, in its infinite wisdom, began to increase the pressure. I didn't know what I wanted to do, so I remained where I was. This time, I didn't have to figure it out. My husband was struggling with his own career. One of the neat side effects of personal growth and healing, is that those around you inevitably begin to grow and change - or flee. Happily, my husband is not a quitter either, and stayed for the adventure. With the pressure off of me, I remained in my comfortably miserable job and focused on supporting him. I put all of the lessons I had learned about the law of attraction to work, and he began to manifest the next step.

It wasn't long before the exact opportunity he was looking for literally fell into his lap. With a push of encouragement from me, we began to figure out the next steps. I am grateful that I couldn't see the path ahead. Had I been able to, I might have run.

I walked into this chapter naively, thinking that he could keep his job and work on his business in his spare time. It didn't take long to realize we were birthing into a much bigger adventure. We outgrew the home we raised our children in and needed a country property to support the growing business. Over the years, we dreamed about returning to the farm life we both grew up in. The timing was never right, the property wasn't quite right, or we couldn't convince a bank that our dreams were worthy. The reality was we weren't ready. We didn't believe, and we didn't know what we wanted.

However, just like magic, and as promised by the Law of Attraction, the perfect place became available the moment we were ready. I had envisioned it years before, described it in detail, and tucked it away in a notebook that held safe my dreams. I had stretched my imagination far enough to believe that I could own it, but my limiting beliefs wouldn't let me see how it was possible.

I dreamed of waking up in that house, walking around in it, and having family dinners in it. I could feel it, I could see us in it. I had no idea how we would afford it, but I knew we were going to live in that house. I felt that home, I lived and breathed that property. We imagined the life we would create. We put in an offer, but financing was denied. We walked away and let the dreams go. However, that home remained, waiting for us. What is meant for you will not pass you by, and 7 months later, we moved in, fully financed, for a fraction of the list price.

We had reached the point in life where we had everything - the country property, the business, and a happy marriage. I had a secret, one that I wasn't prepared to face but I wasn't going to be able to run from. There is nothing like a push to the ground to see where you are. To see how well you have learned the lessons of the past, and how you will move forward. I suspected something was wrong but it was just a feeling. Eventually there was evidence that cancer was beginning to ravish my body.

I was terrified. Cancer took my papa, and I had watched my husband's grandparents both pass away from cancer while I knew it was quietly growing in me. I was angry that this was how my life was going to end, but I didn't want to upset the lives of those around me, so I stayed quiet. I wasn't ready to hear the words, and I was living in a dangerous bubble of denial.

The Universe, in its infinite wisdom, gave me ample opportunity to make a decision, offering me injuries and not so subtle hints about dying. I continued to choose fear, and ignored the disaster I was inviting in. Finally, my own doctor's office called me in for a checkup. I could have made an excuse, and almost left the office without mentioning my very obvious cancer. I chose me in that moment, took a deep breath, and let go of the fear. The weight that lifted off of me that day was incredible. I was scared, but allowing someone else to guide me, to just focus on me was liberating.

This part of the story unfolded as the pandemic was shutting the world down. It was a mixed blessing, I was forced to only look after myself and not worry about anything else. I felt a sense of relief, allowing the doctors to tell me what the course of treatment would be. I needed help, and I needed the chemo boost to get ahead of the cancer.

Initially, it was considered stage 2, possibly stage 3. Thanks to covid, the testing was delayed, and I began treatment within a few days of the diagnosis. It wasn't until the second chemo infusion, that I was told it was stage 4 with metastasis to the bones. I wasn't given a good prognosis. It was here that my innate survival instinct kicked in. It saved my life.

Something was sparked within me that day. It was familiar and primal all at the same time. It was a fire that began to burn as I made a decision to show the oncologist what I could do. I took control of my treatment and used their logic to my advantage. I wanted just enough chemo to shrink the tumors and then surgery. Radiation wasn't on my radar. I wanted to find a balance between what my body needed, and not going overboard. I didn't overthink. I went on instinct and my own internal logic. I dug deep, and got my way, fighting my oncologist's bias and logic, so I got the treatment I knew I needed.

I began to explore alternative and complementary therapies as well. I was focused on my body and mitigating the side effects. I began acupuncture and consulted with a naturopath for supplements that would support the health and repair of my body. I focused on my health and that served me well during active treatment.

I felt remarkable, but after surgery, and after the hair began to grow back, doubt began to set in. Emotions surfaced, and everything that I had ever repressed began to flow out of me. I sank into rock bottom, finally falling through a hole that went well beyond rock bottom. I was lost. I wanted to close my eyes and never wake up again. I was exhausted and couldn't find a way out. I was stuck in a loop and there wasn't a way out.

Until that day under the tree.

A new spark was lit. It was small, a fragile flicker, but it was enough to light the darkness for me to find a way out of the depression I was in. I climbed out, and began a long journey upwards.

I made a decision to live. I realized it was time to create a better version of me, let everything go, and begin to carefully build myself back up. I was tired of being afraid and holding onto the past. I recognized that if I had created the perfect environment within me to allow cancer to grow, I could very likely create an environment it couldn't grow in.

I began to vocally take charge of my treatment. My oncologist was not on board with me, so I began to do my own thing. I wanted to show him that a patient who took control of their journey could have a better outcome than what he had given me, which was "your way will not improve lifespan."

I live with the intention to enjoy every day, even the mundane. Each day is precious, and I am grateful. I envision my future, and while I don't travel too far ahead in my visions, I am enjoying the infinite possibilities. I am not afraid. I forgave myself for how I coped when I didn't know any other way. I am still learning, I still stumble, and occasionally I question myself. I am okay with that. Stepping into your life, and taking responsibility, opens a world of possibility and joy. It is never too late to live.

I'll say it again: Loving who you are, where you are, is the key to living your best life. That's all. Only you can define what that means for you. No one else. Dream, do, live, love!

As I navigate my new reality, I am reminded of how magical life is if you let it show you the way. I have been blessed beyond measure. Life truly is beautiful.

Ann's Story, Part 6

I was making it up to Reno every other week for my intravenous vitamin C infusions until winter of 22-23 hit. I've lived in Mammoth Lakes for twenty-three years, and I've never seen a winter like the one I just lived through.

395, the main north-south highway was closed for weeks at a time, effectively shutting my town off from the rest of the world. I couldn't make it to Reno. Around Christmas time, a couple of local entrepreneurs began offering infusion therapy. One refused to give me 60 grams of IVC, which was my usual dose.

Their max was ten. And they wanted 300 bucks for it. I was paying $375 for 60 grams. *Caveat emptor* is the name of the game here.

The other outfit agreed to my dose, but they didn't mix any buffering agents with the Vitamin C. Also, there are a lot of different Vitamin C formulations out there. I don't believe they used sodium ascorbate, the type utilized in Reno. They also didn't use my port because they didn't have the special needle it required.

Let's just say it wasn't a peak experience. Absent buffering agents, my forearms turned into nine kinds of hell shortly after the infusion began to flow. I threw in the towel after maybe 40 out of 60 grams. They emailed me many times (think cash cow...) but I wasn't interested.

In so many ways my cancer journey has been intuitive.

Remember how I was certain chemotherapy wasn't for me? Genomic testing proved me right.

I stopped feeling guilty about not driving to Reno every two weeks since I couldn't with the road closed. I had two infusions in December, one in January, one in February, one in March, two in April, one in May.

My plan with Dr Devlin was I'd be done in March anyway. After consulting with him, he suggested I continue every four to six weeks for another year. I'm working on it, but my last infusion was 5/8. It's nearing the end of June. Best case scenario, I'll get back there in July since I'm out of the area on an extended road trip.

I'm not sure how critical more IVC is at this point. I had something like twenty-five infusions. Referring to the Riordan Clinic's website (they're the "experts" on IVC) their recommendation is about that number of infusions total.

After struggling and suffering with my port for basically the entire time I had it, I made an appointment to have it removed at my local hospital at the end of March 2023 roughly thirteen months after I'd had it placed.

Removal didn't go much smoother than any other part of the port process, but the local interventional radiologist and his team were rockstars: competent and caring. In fact, the entire Radiology department is stellar. Now that I'm almost three months out from the surgical procedure to rid myself of it, I'm finally healing. For a while suture material was extruding through my skin. My body never has been good at dissolving "dissolvable" stitches.

I've always been jealous of those people whose ports never bothered them, but they weren't out shoveling snow for three months straight multiple times a day. The dry, light powder Mammoth Lakes is famous for failed to make an appearance this year. What fell out of the sky was wet and heavy. So heavy I had to take chunks out of the drifts I shoveled because if I'd taken an entire top-to-bottom shovelful, I wouldn't have been able to lift it. And then there was the problem of volume. The snow was so far above the railing of the UPPER decks, I had to have my husband push it toward the neighbor's house because I couldn't throw shovelfuls that high.

When we left for our road trip on May 20th, the house was still surrounded by ten foot snowbanks.

Enough about snow. My point was that cancer's not the only thing that sets the stage for post-traumatic stress.

Meanwhile, protocol for uterine cancers like mine is gynecologic visits every three months for the first two years.

Toward that end, the Stanford MD had moved to southern California because her husband (also an MD) got an important job down there. She invited me to follow her. Interestingly, southern California is way more convenient for me than the Bay Area. It's a straight shot driving south without any major mountain passes once I leave home.

I made my first trek down there in August 2022. And I saw my doctor and a resident since my doctor was teaching faculty for UCLA's OB-GYN residency program. The place I saw her was a clinic run by the County of Los Angeles. I was about the only native English speaker there, but it was fine so long as I got time with an MD I'd come to value.

Push the clock forward to November. After another 700-mile round trip, I saw a resident. My doctor wasn't there. I messaged her through the patient portal to ask if she was still my doctor. She reassured me she was and promised to be there for my next appointment.

February 2023 rolled around. Another long drive to the LA County Clinic. This time, I didn't even see an MD. They shunted me to a nurse practitioner. I'm far from a snob, but that pretty much did it.

The MD I'd driven all that way to see didn't even have the courtesy to let me know she wouldn't be there. Out of all my MD woes, that rejection really hurt. I'd been under the illusion she actually cared about me, but apparently she was just going through the motions.

There wasn't much point in further visits to Sylmar, so I retreated to the OB-GYN I'd established care with in Bishop and scheduled my May quarterly visit with her. I like her very much, and she was empathetic about the ex-Stanford MD ghosting me.

I'm now on an every-six-month schedule for exams.

Have I just had bad luck with MDs? I don't think so.

Practicing medicine isn't as satisfying as it once was. MDs invited the twin devils of Big Pharma and insurance companies into what was once a sacrosanct relationship between them and their patients. The result has been pretty ugly. Doctors are leaving the field in unprecedented numbers.

Finding a new one is tough.

Getting an appointment with old ones is too.

According to Dr. Devlin, 85 percent of recurrences happen in the first two years with aggressive cancers. I feel mildly relieved to have passed that milestone. Yet I'm far from out of the woods.

Changes I've made in my life in terms of taking handfuls of supplements, making certain to get exercise, and avoiding dairy, grain, processed foods, and sugar will remain hallmarks of my existence for however many more years are granted to me.

My last visit to the OB-GYN in Bishop, her parting words were, "You've come a long way since I first saw you."

I took it as a compliment.

My first visit there was right after my second surgery. I had a Foley catheter draining urine into a bag strapped to my leg and a stent from my right kidney threaded into my bladder. I had a chronic bladder infection from the Foley.

One of the best days of my life was when I showed up at her clinic three weeks to the minute after the Foley was placed to have it removed. The Bishop doc had specific instructions from Dr. Icon, and she followed them to a T.

It still took several weeks for my urinary tract to clear any trace of infection, but at least the plastic tube holding my urethra open was gone.

Once you've heard the words, "You have cancer," you can never un-hear them. Neither can you retreat to your pre-cancer world.

There is always the possibility "it" will resurface.

That surgical screw-up, the one where the surgeon fried my ureter, had a 1 percent chance of occurrence. Cold comfort if you're that 1 percent. Extrapolating, my numbers are better now. 15 percent chance of recurrence is way better than 40 percent, but I remain vigilant.

I've occasionally cheated on the food front, but the guilt is so pervasive, it's not worth it. I don't enjoy food like I used to. Mostly, I look at it as calories I need to keep my weight up. And energy for daily exercise. I have altered my baking to create things I can eat, but part of me will always miss the decadence of fudge or ice cream or pecan pie.

Not that I ever ate a lot of anything like that. But in the olden days, I could. Now they're definitely off the table.

None of this is easy, but avoiding sugar is a small sacrifice to pay. Avoiding alcohol is simple since I never enjoyed anything beyond a few sips of microbrewed beer.

I'm alive, and grateful for every damned second of my life. When that long ago doc—the one who had no idea where to refer me—dropped the bombshell words, I was certain I was a dead woman walking.

I'm far from alone in my feelings. The other survivor stories in this book offer a snapshot of their journeys. There are many points of concordance. Nearly everyone engages in exercise, some type of meditation, a specific diet, and certain supplements.

Taking responsibility for one's own care is a hallmark. Doctors are advisors, nothing more or less.

I dithered back and forth about replacing the gynecologic oncologist who ghosted me. In the end, I decided not to. For one thing, they'd demand I go to them for my biannual visits. It would mean more long drives. I'd much rather go to Bishop to an MD I know and respect.

Starting over with new doctors is difficult. I'm past assuming someone will be a wonderful human being who went into medicine because of a pervasive desire to do good in the world. That's far truer of subspecialties like family medicine, pediatrics, and psychiatry. Ophthalmologists and dermatologists and plastic surgeons are a cheery crew, but I don't need their services.

I would approach a new care provider with some level of trepidation. It would bleed through, and we'd be off to a sketchy start from the gate.

My fond hope is I never have to go there.

A few more chapters will round out this book. Another survivor story. A discussion of the importance of supporting our spiritual sides as we heal. One on integrative oncology, another on nutrition.

Kudos to you if you hung in there and are still reading.

Dan Lyster's Story

DAN LYSTER'S PROSTATE CANCER JOURNEY

As told to Stacey Lyster

Note from Ann: Dan and Stacey are my neighbors. In Mammoth Lakes, that means more than it might elsewhere. For one thing, this is a very small community. Winters are harsh, and we help one another. Years ago, Dan and I both worked for Mono County. He was the county "Energy Czar," and I ran the mental health department.

In August 2016 I went up to a urologist in Carson City after my general practitioner, Dr. Clark, said my PSA count was higher than usual. He said the numbers were above the normal PSA. It was 4.99. He said I could continue to watch it or I could have a biopsy for some peace of mind.

I met with Dr. Nixon, the urologist in Carson City. He did the biopsy of my prostate. After waiting two weeks I went in to see him with my wife, Stacey. I never thought I had prostate cancer, but the waiting was still difficult. Turns out I had two small tumors in my prostate. We both sat there in shock. Seeing I was visibly upset, my wife put her arms around me. I immediately thought of my cousin and a few other people who had prostate cancer and who had decided to have their prostates removed. They seemed to be doing okay, even with their side effects. I didn't see it as an immediate death sentence and started my journey to see what I was going to do to get rid of the cancer. Stacey's dad died of prostate cancer, so she was a bit freaked out and wanted the thing out of me as soon as possible. And now her husband had prostate cancer, so she was ultra-sensitive about the fact that I had the same thing. I think she said something like, "I don't give a fuck if we have sex anymore. I want you alive."

I started researching my options. I made an appointment with a surgeon at Stanford to talk about the robotic removal of the prostate. I also went to another doctor in Reno who used Cyberknife where they use a laser to attack the tumors. I read about Cryo-therapy as well.

Somewhere along the line my stepson, Erik, told me about Rick Simpson oil, which is a condensed version of THC cannabis oil that can be made into suppositories. I did research online about the effects of cannabis on cancer cells. Additionally, Stacey's cousin, Jeff, gave me a cancer protocol to use because his mother had pancreatic cancer and when she was vigilant about using the protocol, her pancreatic cancer numbers started to decline. As soon as she started to eat sugar and flour again, her pancreatic cancer metastasized and she eventually passed away. My decision was to do "Active Surveillance" along with the Rick Simpson oil and the cancer protocol. Stacey was not happy, but it was my decision.

I started taking 30 tablets a day of Wobenzym. According to Stacey's cousin, the theory was that Wobenzym will begin to shrink existing tumors and prevent the cancer from metastasizing. Enzymes erode the fibrin (outside shell) of the cancer cells. I also started doing a green juice every day. My counter looked like one of the shelves in a health food store. I would add kale, parsley, cilantro, cucumber, spinach, and celery. Everything had to be organic. Adding organic beets and small doses of turmeric were also recommended.

I added 10,000 units of Vitamin D3 and K2 which also help prevent the spread of cancer. I added 16 grams of Chaga mushrooms and the IP6 supplement which has been proven to reduce cancer by shortening the life of cancer cells.

I tried to stop eating any and all flesh foods and absolutely no dairy. The hardest thing was for me to stop drinking milk. I had been drinking a gallon of milk every two days since I was a kid for about 60 years. According to the cancer protocol, almost all milk products in the United States contain Bovine Growth Hormones (BGH). It's not listed as an ingredient but it's present. BGH causes cancer and has been banned in many countries, but is still legal in the U.S. All milk products contain casein, a phyto-protein that has been found in numerous studies to exacerbate cancer growth. It has been said that dairy may speed up the growth of cancer cells and in some cases, activate the growth mechanism for dormant cancer cells.

I started making my own suppositories and used them once a day for two months. I continued to monitor my PSA every six months. The first time I went in for an MRI of my prostate after I was diagnosed, it showed some suspect areas but couldn't pinpoint exactly what was going on or where the tumors were. My PSA had gone up to 5.9 so I continued to use the suppositories, gave up dairy, and then I had an MRI-guided biopsy a year after the diagnosis. They had a hard time detecting the tumors. My doctor said that the cancer was not gone but it was so small they couldn't see the tumors they saw when I was first diagnosed. I continued to do the same protocol and a year later I had another MRI at the hospital where I live in Mammoth Lakes. My GP said he talked it over with his colleagues and even though there were still suspicious areas, nothing seemed to be metastatic or carcinogenic in the results.

Six months later I talked again with my urologist. He said he couldn't explain it and was convinced the cancer was still there somewhere. He wanted to do another needle biopsy, guided by an ultrasound. He did that in his office and when I met with him he said, "Well, you've had two back-to-back needle biopsies that haven't revealed any cancer so I have to give you a clean bill of health." He said in his experience this had never happened, but he wasn't ready to say that anything I had been doing had been responsible for getting rid of the cancer. That was in 2019. It's now 2023 and to the best of my knowledge I am still cancer free.

Spiritual Pursuits

According to standard of care oncology, we are only bodies, our physical selves. It's the sole aspect most oncologists treat. We are far more multifaceted than that because we are body, mind, emotions, and spirit. Everything needs to be in sync, which means we have to develop awareness of all the parts of ourselves.

Most of us have a strong side, one we lead with. For athletes, it's their bodies. Professors probably lead with their minds. Actors may lead with emotions. Regardless, discovering our individual strength and playing to it is important, as is developing our less prominent aspects.

One thread that runs through many survivor stories is mention of a crossroads where the individual decided to stop doing things they found unpalatable and developed the backbone to stand up for themselves and say no.

We cannot be whole until we do that, until we own who we are and can unashamedly stand before the world without mouthing excuses.

It's not accidental that nearly every cancer book I've read, and every survivor story, has highlighted the importance of our spiritual sides as they relate to healing. By spiritual, I do not necessarily mean religious, although those with a strong religious background can certainly leverage it to aid in healing.

Fair warning, those with traditional religious leanings may feel the rest of this chapter offers short shrift for their beliefs. Nothing could be further from the truth. The critical element is belief in a higher power. I honor every path people choose.

For me, spiritual pursuits engender giving up the illusion of control. That's a hard one for me. If my psychologist is reading this, he's laughing his head off since I've always been a control queen.

Additionally, it means accepting something larger than us is out there, no matter how we envision it. Every successful healing story incorporates spirituality on some level.

The mountains are my spiritual home. Traipsing through the backcountry is where I learned to believe in myself. I've spent a lot of time alone with a pack on my back on- and off-trail. Particularly the winter backcountry, with its expansive vistas of white, pounds home how truly small and insignificant I am in the grand scheme of things.

It's not a bad thing since it provides perspective. Problems that were insurmountable feel far less daunting. Find your own magical spot, one where simply being there brings you peace. It can be as simple as a special chair in your home or a steaming bath.

No rights or wrongs here.

Many moons ago when I was at university, the Carlos Castaneda books were in vogue. Part of the message in those books, which borrowed heavily from Eastern philosophers, was to live as if Death sat on one shoulder. In other words, conduct yourself in such a way that if you dropped dead, you'd have nothing to apologize for and no regrets.

Also during my university days, I was Charles Tart's teaching assistant. He was one of the original altered states of consciousness researchers and introduced me to the work of the Russian philosopher Georges Gurdjieff. Dr. Tart hosted an intriguing bunch of visitors like Baba Ram Dass, Rolling Thunder, and a few others. I learned to meditate back then and kept it up for a number of years, but life intervened.

One of cancer's gifts—and there have been many—is it offered an opportunity to resurrect my badly neglected meditation practice. In her story, Maria closes with mentioning she's happier and healthier now than she was before she heard the words, "You have cancer."

This disease does have gifts. Finding and articulating them is one tool to support your health and well-being.

There are so many paths to still your mind, to quiet the incessant chatter telling you to do this, that, or the other thing. Or worse, predicting gloom and doom because you failed to do something. I used to tell my patients to live in the moment. It's easy to say, much tougher to do.

Today is the tomorrow you worried about yesterday...

Take a few moments to think about that.

What happened yesterday is done. What's going to happen tomorrow isn't here yet. When we focus on the now, it's powerful. When we meditate or pray, we are present, not worried about what we should have done. Sometimes we get sidetracked, but then we come back to the breath. It's a constant, always with us.

Soothing if we allow it to be. Our breath is like coming home to ourselves. One of the simplest of meditations is thinking, "I am" when you inhale, and "home" on the exhale.

Every time I sit to meditate doesn't yield relaxation. Sometimes I can't quiet my mind, but there's always next time. The critical part is consistency and avoiding an all-too-human tendency to criticize less-than-perfect efforts. I meditate in the morning to set the stage for my day, and again before bed to rid myself of any residual anxiety. I also do Wim Hoff breathing and cold immersion in the morning. The latter has become easier even through our long winters.

Beyond meditation, there are martial arts, other types of structured breathing, Qi Gong, Zen sound bath, Reiki, Buddhist practices, and ever so many others. You Tube is a veritable treasure trove of all the above.

Similar to exercise, the key is finding something that sings to your soul, something you can do every day, something you look forward to as a shining island of peace.

Stress initiates a cascade of hormones that keeps our bodies in a state of perpetual arousal. That state isn't conducive to healing anything. Chronic stress can set the stage for the development of cancer and other serious diseases.

Many of the survivor stories in this book highlight a stressor— or a string of them—that presaged their diagnosis. We cannot avoid stress, but we can mitigate our response to it.

Not trying to harp on meditation, but it's a simple tool that requires no cash outlay and can be practiced anywhere. No matter what we run up against, taking a few moments to breathe will make it more palatable. The same holds for prayer. You can pray anywhere.

Because cancer is a long-term proposition, every survivor needs to cultivate tools to settle their emotions when the "what if it comes back" demons come out to play.

And they will.

It happens to all of us. Those who've internalized skills to acknowledge difficult thoughts and allow them to wash over and through them tend to fare better.

For me, this is where integrative oncology truly shines. It espouses a whole patient approach, not just surgery, chemo, and radiation. This is also where group support is important. They did social psychology studies years ago that proved the illusion of social support is just as potent as actual social support.

Enter the Internet. As you join integrative care support groups and become active in them, you'll find a valuable network, even though you'll probably never meet any of the people involved. Many reside in different countries.

They all have something in common, though. They understand where you're at because they've been there too.

Find a spiritual pursuit you can stick with. It might not be the first one you try, or even the second. Eventually, something will sing to your heart and soul. That's the modality for you. Carve out daily time to nurture your spirit. It's as important to your healing as anything else you do.

Let's move on to nutrition.

Nutrition

I'd toyed with writing a chapter on nutrition. It's so important addressing cancer there are literally hundreds—possibly thousands—of books devoted to the topic. Against that backdrop, it felt pretentious for me to even try to tackle it, but then writing this book at all was so far out of my comfort zone, what's one more chapter?

Two things happened when I thought I was done with *Alive*. One of my contributors dropped out at the last minute. Another contributor sent me a fascinating article titled, *Dietary Interventions and Precision Nutrition in Cancer Therapy*. The investigators were Carlos Martinez-Garay and Nabil Djouder, Ph.D. The article can be found in the July 2023 edition of Trends in Molecular Medicine (29/7), pages 489-511.

If I've learned anything through this cancer saga, it's been to go with the flow and trust things happen for reasons. I suddenly had space in the book to add the chapter I'd been considering. I solicited one more story from a woman I'd met months ago, and I decided to attempt to expand on the topic of nutrition, something I've touched on throughout this book.

Obviously, I won't cover all the bases—or even a majority of them. How could I? What comes next is merely a starting point.

Highlights from *Dietary Interventions and Precision Nutrition in Cancer Therapy* discuss new studies that are finally proving what we take into our bodies can have a radical effect on whether we get cancer in the first place, and what happens to existing cancers when we continue to consume a sub-optimal diet. The article stresses that cancers are as unique as the people who get the disease; thus, a precision approach is necessary. One which tailors food (and supplements) to each individual and their condition.

I found their research refreshing and exciting because it stresses something I've suspected for years: we are what we eat. It's an uphill battle to either be healthy, or regain health, when we exist on highly processed foods because they're convenient.

We're busier than our parents. Far busier than our grandparents. Those generations could afford to have one adult in the home preparing meals and perhaps gardening and canning. Today's economics make it much harder to not have everyone in a household (except children) gainfully employed. The way we've compensated is by substituting take-out, frozen, and other pre-prepared meal items because no one has the energy to peel, chop, sauté, bake, or roast. Not on a 365 days/year basis.

The other phenomenon, as the world has grown smaller, is produce and meat from other countries are flown in. Never mind the carbon footprint aspect of that. Unless produce is grown organically, it's treated to allow it to retain an (artificial) freshness through long hours in an airplane. The same is true for meats. When I purchase, for example, lamb that was raised in Australia I wonder how "organic" it actually is. A good rule of thumb is the closer a foodstuff is to its native environment, the better it is for you. So a peach, hopefully organically grown, has far more nutrients the moment it's picked than it will have by the time we purchase it from our local supermarket.

Compounding this problem is the fact that commercial growers want their products to survive transport, so they pick them while they're still "green." I'm sure you've all had the experience of bringing hard-as-rocks peaches home, only to have them rot before they become edible. Those peaches lack the nutrient composition of a peach allowed to ripen naturally.

Sometimes, it seems like the food industry is trying to kill us, when all they're after is making a profit.

If there are farmer's markets in your area, they're a decent source of fresher produce. Also, many small ranches exist where you can purchase grass-fed beef and free-range chicken.

The journal article I led out with addresses specific diets. It covers the topics of calorie restriction (intermittent fasting and longer fasting), ketogenic diets, the Mediterranean diet, and fast mimicking diets. The article sits behind a paywall, but the fee to read it is reasonable. In the 3.99 USD range. It is technical in nature, and it will not tell you which foods or supplements to either eat or avoid, but the research aspect is intriguing, and it's well-referenced.

At least in theory, now that we have the technology to do molecular and/or genomic testing on tumors and our bodies, we have access to a wealth of data. Included is what type of metabolism drives our particular cancers—and us. Once we have those pieces of data, we can select an eating plan to hopefully effectively starve cancer.

One of the issues with that approach is cancer is a sneaky beast. A cancer that was very happy living on glucose, will grudgingly switch to fatty acids if its glucose supply is cut off. Or to glutamine. What that means is being vigilant, checking labs and other relevant indicators for alterations in the status quo.

We find ways to live with cancer, but we never "get over" it.

Jane McLelland was truly a pioneer in this field. A cancer survivor herself, she refused to allow recurrences to turn into a death sentence. Her research about mapping pathways based on mutations has been one of the cornerstones for an entire field addressing cancer's metabolic pathways. Because her work targeted a lay audience, it engendered wide appeal.

One of my initial visits with the integrative oncologist yielded a glucometer, finger prick needles, and test strips. My task was to monitor my blood glucose levels. Long before that, I'd conferred with my PCP, and we'd started me on metformin, a glucose-lowering agent used for type-2 diabetics. I have never been diabetic, but I started metformin, anyway. Among other things, it was identified as a potent anti-aging supplement back in the 1980s.

Getting used to Metformin wasn't a simple task. That drug isn't especially pleasant. It took me about a month to build up to where I could tolerate 500 mgs. At that point, I switched to the extended-release version and increased my dose to two a day. Once I was convinced my blood glucose was stable, and within Dr. Devlin's recommended limits, I stopped checking so often. The whole process gave me a fresh appreciation for diabetics. You only have so many fingers, and the place you prick them gets sore.

Later on, and with help, I mapped mutational pathways identified from two places. I used Nutrition Genome (a saliva test) for my body genomics, and CARIS for my tumor genomics. The results yielded a significant change in my daily supplement regimen.

This will be an individual endeavor for each of you. Another test, NutrEval from Genova Diagnostics, also provides a genetic snapshot of your body genomics. It's available through practitioners and uses blood and urine. It's more accurate than Nutrition Genome. Both tests suggest foods that are compatible with your unique makeup.

As I noted elsewhere, we all got cancer for a reason. One of the simplest things we can alter is how we eat and the supplements we take. I'm not sure how it is outside of the U.S., but it's not easy to obtain quality food throughout this country.

Where I live, not much is available that's labeled USDA organic. Finding grass fed meat or wild caught seafood is a crapshoot. Not that I consume dairy products anymore, but I have noticed the dairy section consistently stocks grassfed milk, which is a big improvement.

What's the big deal about grassfed, anyway? Grassfed dairy has more omega-3 fatty acids. This is important because Western diets are high in omega-6s and low in omega-3s, resulting in an imbalanced ratio of about 15:1. This is partly due to the excessive consumption of highly processed foods and limited consumption of fish, along with added seed and vegetable oils in the Western diet.

Since I brought up oils, a while back I mentioned to someone that I was making pancakes with toasted walnut oil. I was firmly reminded to only fry with avocado or olive oils. They should be organic and cold-pressed. Oils processed with heat and stored in plastic bottles are potentially carcinogenic. Avoid refined oils at all times.

Reading labels is paramount. You'd be surprised how many grocery items have added sugar: nearly all of them from salad dressing to marinara sauce. The best answer I came up with was making everything myself, which is time-consuming.

Someone going through chemotherapy and/or radiation needs access to healthy food requiring minimal preparation. If it's not available, the fallback to processed food isn't helpful.

Food is comfort for some of us. Restrictions aren't palatable. Cancer is a disease of losses. If a major dietary alteration isn't in the cards, try deleting one thing. If you've mapped your mutations, pick the top-of-the list item and make a commitment to (mostly) avoid it.

Since so many cancers are glucose-driven, the first food item to scratch off the list is sugar. You can still have Manuka honey, organic maple syrup, and coconut sugar (lower glycemic index), but in SMALL quantities. And not every day. It will take time for a palate used to uber-sweet foods to adjust, but it's doable.

Soda is one more place where it's simple to stop drinking them. The "regular ones" are chock full of sugar from high fructose corn syrup. The diet version isn't good for you, either. Mineral water with a small splash of fruit juice can be a reasonable substitute.

As long as I mentioned water, it's critical too. Buy a decent water filter. Whole house ones are perfect. Failing that, at least filter your drinking and cooking water. Don't forget the shower. Skin is your body's largest organ. Contaminants can soak in through it. There are many showerhead/filter combos on the market. Be sure to purchase additional filters and change them regularly.

The other food-related topic is cookware. All the glitzy nonstick pans should be avoided. The nonstick coating breaks down over time when exposed to high heat, and it has carcinogenic properties. I'm also not fond of microwaves. Never, never microwave food wrapped in plastic in the microwave. No Styrofoam, either. Replace all that nonstick cookware and aluminum with stainless steel or cast iron. Additionally, store your food in glass or aluminum foil, not plastic.

Toward the back of her book, *The Metabolic Approach to Cancer*, Nasha Winters has a comprehensive section about overhauling your kitchen, so what you eat and the utensils you cook with support your health rather than tearing it down. The book is worth its purchase price for that section alone.

Let's take a quick look at specialized diets starting with calorie restriction. This can be a slippery slope for those who are too thin to start with, although interestingly, experiments with calorie restriction haven't pushed the "too thin" into an anorexic range. Calorie restriction is a time-honored anti-aging method.

As noted by Greg in his story, anything that's good for anti-aging is also good for anti-cancer.

There's out-and-out fasting where you do a water fast for, perhaps, one or two days every couple of weeks. Some fast one day a week. Some fast two days every couple of weeks. Fasting for more than three days at a stretch reverses the benefits. Taking care with the refeeding period after a fast is important. There are many resources that can lead you through the process.

Intermittent fasting yields almost the same benefits. This includes limiting your eating to a specific window each day with a 15-18 hours break between the evening meal and the morning one. Recent research suggests 13 hours is a better "sweet spot," but the jury is still out on that one.

Then there is a fast-mimicking diet. This consists of high fat, some protein, and very low carbs. It's practiced in five-day stretches about once a month. Valter Longo has pre-built kits you can buy from him and also Fast Bars, a type of nutritional bar. They aren't bad. I have several boxes left over from my brief stint with chemo.

A few preliminary human trials have shown a decrease in risk for cancer or a decrease in cancer growth rates with fasting. These studies indicate this may be due to the following effects:

- decreased blood glucose production
- stem cells triggered to regenerate the immune system
- balanced nutritional intake
- increased production of tumor-killing cells

In one study of time-restricted feeding during 9–12 hour phases, fasting was shown to reverse the progression of obesity and type-2 diabetes in mice. Obesity is a major risk factor for cancer, which may support fasting to treat it.

A second study using mice showed that a bimonthly fast-mimicking diet reduced the incidence of cancer. Results were similar in a pilot trial with nineteen humans by the same scientists. It showed decreased biomarkers and risk factors for cancer.

In a 2016 study, research showed that a combination of fasting and chemotherapy slowed the progression of breast cancer and skin cancer. The combined treatment methods caused the body to produce higher levels of common lymphoid progenitor cells (CLPs) and tumor-infiltrating lymphocytes. CLPs are the precursor cells to lymphocytes, which are white blood cells that migrate into a tumor and are known for killing tumors.

The same study noted short-term starvation makes cancer cells sensitive to chemotherapy while protecting normal cells, and it also promoted the production of stem cells.

Leaving the topic of fasting, the Mediterranean diet features lots of fresh fruit and vegetables, whole grains, fish, beans, olive oil, and nuts. It's one of the simplest eating plans to follow because of the variety.

Ketogenic diets work on the theory that you eat mostly fat with limited protein and almost no carbohydrates. It pushes your body into ketogenesis, where you're burning fat for fuel rather than glucose. This diet can be tough, particularly the cancer version which doesn't include bacon, cheese, and the other items that are hallmarks of a "regular" keto eating plan. Also, the composition of non-carbohydrate macronutrients in a ketogenic diet is important. Adaptations to carbohydrate-restricted diets can create compensatory reactions. Certain amino acid combinations can actually form glucose. Therefore, the amino acid composition of these diets has to be carefully monitored.

There are simple ways to check for ketosis. You can order urine test strips from several online retailers. Between those and a simple glucometer, you can stay on top of whether your eating plan is doing what you hope it is.

Assistance is helpful in choosing which of these eating plans is the right one for you and your cancer. Naturopaths and nutritionists, who specialize in cancer, can be extraordinarily helpful. Integrative oncologists, too.

If you lack access to help determining how to move forward, a strong first step is intermittent fasting and eliminating sugar and processed foods from your diet. It's not easy. Well, the sugar part was for me, but processed foods, e.g. things like Amy's frozen entrees, are convenience items.

I enjoy cooking, but not every night. Sometimes, the creative well runs dry. Those of you who live in large urban areas have restaurants serving unprocessed, healthy food. I wish I did.

Just as everyone's cancer is different, so is everyone's living situation. The other food-linked problem is that suddenly your diet is different from everyone else's in the family—unless they simply go along with whatever you're eating. This means making separate menu items, not the easiest endeavor on a day-in, day-out basis.

I've been fortunate that my energy has been decent except around my two surgeries. Many people with cancer don't have the extra energy it takes to turn out multiple meals every day. It's not just cooking. It's shopping and meal planning. See if you can enlist help from friends and family.

I am encouraged that food—and supplements—are finally topics being studied by researchers. None of the oncologists I saw said boo about food. It's as if they didn't see any connection between what we eat and cancer progression. The integrative oncologist, however, stressed food. He wanted to know what I was eating, and he was quite clear what to steer clear of. As an interesting sidenote, he's part owner of a natural food restaurant.

Concluding remarks from the article noted at the beginning of this chapter stress that we finally have the technology to move away from generalized "one size fits all" cancer treatment to personalized interventions based on microbiome screening, molecular/genomic tests, and nutrigenomics. Against that backdrop, they envision a future where precision nutrition will be a preferred therapeutic approach. Part of this strategy will include specific diets developed based on metabolism, disease state, pre-existing conditions, and safety.

These researchers are located in Madrid at the Spanish National Cancer Center. Perhaps things have shifted there to treating patients based on molecular/genomic profiles, but the shift hasn't yet found its way to the U.S., where many of us have to beg for genomic testing. It's far from a given.

Regardless of feasibility in this country, I find their premise—and conclusions—captivating and promising. We have come a long way from the days when Jane McLelland, relentless pioneer attempting to save her own life—which she did—embarked on her solo journey researching how she could make her body an inhospitable environment for cancer. She got a few things wrong, but she got a whole lot right. More importantly, she paved the way for the rest of us to ask questions and not accept our diagnoses as death sentences.

Change is more palatable when taken in small chunks. Start with one thing. Add others over time. Find a reputable naturopath and a nutritionist. Add an integrative oncologist to the mix. Many of them do telehealth or phone visits, so you're not limited by geography. Nasha Winters, ND, an ovarian cancer survivor, lists practitioners she's trained on her website.

It's a decent starting point. So is the list of Facebook groups in the Resource section. Someone in one of them will live in your geographic area and will have ideas about who you can see.

To continue eating the way you were before your diagnosis is akin to playing roulette. Since none of us will ever know why "it" happened to us, it makes sense to hedge our bets.

Moving on to integrative oncology.

Integrative Oncology

What is integrative oncology, anyway?

If you look at the Mayo Clinic definition, you'll find it's adjunctive interventions used alongside conventional ones. If you take a peek at Andrew Weil, you'll find lifestyle changes are key to dealing with any disease entity.

If you ask most traditional oncologists, they'll discount anything except their cut, burn, and poison approach. This circles back to the sugar laden junk food so prevalent at infusion centers. Obesity is a significant risk factor for many diseases including cancer. Oncologists have a golden opportunity to teach their patients the value of a healthy lifestyle, but they usually fail to do so for reasons I theorized earlier in this book.

Beyond my theories, nutrition isn't part of most medical school curricula.

My take on integrative oncology, or integrative anything with a health focus, is that it takes a village. Our physical bodies are inextricably linked to our minds, emotions, and spirits.

It's well-documented that stress feeds cancer, sets the stage for disease to develop. It also nurtures existing disease, worsening it.

It makes sense that we need to focus on healing the whole person. When we do that, we have a decent chance of maximizing our true selves. In their stories, Lena makes the point that the whole "battling cancer" concept is antithetical to healing. Going to war against yourself isn't productive.

Earlier in this book, I mentioned that my psychologist said much the same thing. He told me I needed to make friends with the cancer, establish détente with it.

The only way out is through. That is true for damn near everything. We don't get to skate out from under the bad stuff that falls into our laps.

One of my favorite stories about Carl Jung is a dream he had. It was a dark and stormy night. The wind was howling; a storm raged around him. This was back in the early 1900s, and so he wore a long topcoat and was sheltering a lantern between his hands. In the dream, he knew he couldn't let its light go out.

Soon, he felt something closing from behind him, a presence that sent chills down his spine. He walked faster, and then began to run. The presence kept pace. Jung was gasping for breath, shaking, and terrified. Finally, he couldn't run anymore, so he stopped and turned around.

What he faced was his shadow. As soon as he did that, his fears dropped away, and the lantern flame burned strongly. We all have a shadow side. It's the parts of us we're ashamed of, the pieces we do our damnedest to hide from the world.

The modern nomenclature for shadow is baggage. We all have some. The question is what we do with those less-than-perfect parts.

Somehow, we have to first own and then integrate them, or we'll never be whole. There are theories out there that all diseases feed on stress. Something about the glucocorticoid cascade keeps the body in a hyperactive state. If we remain hypervigilant for days, weeks, months, years, it takes a serious toll.

What's needed is inner peace.

Whole different focus from "kicking cancer's ass."

How can we do that when the cancer is part of us? We'd be kicking ourselves, scarcely a productive pursuit.

That was long-winded. Circling back to integrative oncology, in my world it's something different for every patient with cancer. Still, common threads run through it. Various intravenous drips—Vitamin C, mistletoe, artesunate, and others—are usually a part of integrative care. Hyperbaric oxygen therapy, ozone therapy, insulin potentiated chemotherapy (very low dose, nontoxic), hyperthermia, PEMF, red light therapy, psychotherapy, and photon therapy are a few interventions.

Hopefully, a reputable clinic will build on those elements, and others, to craft a unique program for each patient.

In addition to the tools offered by integrative oncology, other life-affirming practices include:

1. Spiritual practices, which encompass anything from organized religion to meditation to breathing practices to being one with nature—and beyond. The hallmark is belief in something beyond yourself and a willingness to give up needing to control every aspect of every day.
2. Consider starting a daily gratitude journal. Write down five things you were grateful for every day before going to bed.
3. Eastern practices like yoga, qi gong, martial arts, acupuncture, and reiki can center us.
4. Food. Some say vegan is the key. Others insist on whole food plant based. Some push keto. So long as an eating plan has a relatively low glycemic index and avoids sugar, processed food, and inflammatory foods, there's a wide range of acceptable possibilities. The next chapter delves into nutrition in greater detail.
5. Intermittent fasting, which restricts food consumption within an eight-to-ten-hour window out of twenty-four, allows your immune system to reset each day. Newer research highlights thirteen hours as the "sweet spot" for this practice.
6. Exercise is key. And this means far more than a leisurely half-hour stroll. You really need to get your heart rate up and sweat for at least 60-90 minutes

several times a week. Start slow if you must but get up and move.
7. Social connections are also important. Loving and being loved are a critical part of healing.
8. A far infrared sauna can help sweat out toxins. It can also clear chemotherapy chemicals from your body. Daily rebound training supports a healthy lymphatic system.

Supplements are important, but regimens have to be developed individually in conjunction with a nutritionist or naturopath or someone who understands the concept of mapping mutations and building a supplement program predicated on your unique needs.

In order to map mutations, you need to have genomic/molecular testing done.

Isn't it interesting how recovering your health hinges on something most standard of care oncologists ignore until a patient's cancer has returned? Then, they might recommend genomic testing to determine next steps.

In my world view, you start with genomics—or a place like Dr. Nagourney's clinic in Long Beach, California. If everyone did, there would be far fewer recurrences.

I take a lot of supplements. Some days, I can't face swallowing one more pill or drinking another shot of modified citrus pectin, so I give myself mini breaks, but then I get back to it. Supplements are my medicine. They're just as potent—and far less toxic—than oral or IV chemotherapies.

Belief plays a strong role too. If you don't have faith in alternative/integrative care, then it's not the path for you. The mind is incredibly powerful. If you view integrative oncology as one step up from voodoo, by all means stick with what you're doing.

One of my observations from the various integrative care cancer groups I belong to is so many members "found" integrative care after traditional care failed them and they were dying.

Integrative care doesn't save everyone. Far from it. But it has a decent track record, at least as good as traditional care without the horrible side effect profile. Chemo and radiation might kill circulating tumor cells, but they also create havoc in the body. Chemo can cause severe neuropathy that doesn't resolve. It also sets the stage for cancer stem cells (remember them?) to proliferate.

I'm sure there are many instances where chemotherapy is useful, but its use needs to be far more individualized than it is currently. I ended up on the receiving end of, "we give everyone with your cancer X and Y." And I am eternally grateful my poor body only had to deal with two infusions rather than six before I discovered X and Y weren't effective in my case.

On other fronts, right after my cancer diagnosis, my PCP prescribed Celexa, an SSRI antidepressant. I broke the first pill in half and spent a miserable few hours viewing my life through a barrier standing between me and experiencing my emotions. I never took another one. Win, lose, or draw, my choice is to experience my life fully no matter how uncomfortable I am.

This is not to say antidepressants are "bad." They simply aren't for me. They do work for many people, but they were designed as a stopgap to allow people to develop coping mechanisms, not as something to take daily for years.

One phenomenon I saw frequently in my psychotherapy practice was what I called, "Fix me, but don't make me change." The upshot was, "Give me a pill." Oftentimes the doctor did, but pills aren't a panacea. Comes a time when you have to take a good hard look at whatever the problem is.

Kicking the can down the road only works for so long.

A whole lot of people have figured out how to live with cancer. We had no choice. Living with cancer sure as hell beats dying from it. Most of us manage by instituting major lifestyle changes. My post-cancer diagnosis morning routine takes roughly two hours. It includes stretching, floor exercises, yoga, Wim Hoff breathing, meditation, rebounding, and kettlebells.

Since I do intermittent fasting, those two hours divert me from being hungry and wanting breakfast. By the time I'm done with everything listed above, it's time for the supplements I take prior to food. When they're done, I work on making breakfast, which happens around ten.

Not that I'm holding myself up as a shining example of, well, anything. But my routine holds commonalities with most cancer survivors who've adopted an integrative path. In many ways, it's much harder than just showing up for chemo and/or radiation and not doing anything further. Some people get away with not instituting any changes in their life prior, during, or after standard of care treatment. Many do not.

Consistency is the key to damn near everything.

Humans are infinitely capable of adjusting to circumstances.

Earlier in this book, I mentioned people get cancer for a variety of reasons. If the only thing you change post diagnosis is doing surgery/chemo/radiation, you're not doing yourself any favors.

You can certainly accept standard of care oncology treatment. I'd never suggest anyone go against an MD's advice unless they felt strongly about it. Still, nowhere is it written you can't institute comprehensive, global changes to support a new, healthier you in conjunction with standard of care treatments.

Several survivor stories in *Alive* blend standard of care with integrative techniques. Each of us determines our own path. To do that, we must become the protagonist in our personal journey.

Get second opinions. Third opinions. Fourth opinions. Keep after it until you're satisfied. Talk with practitioners from different persuasions. Forge your own path. Believe in your body's innate ability to heal.

I have no idea what the future holds for me, but I hope I have the ability to face it with grace and dignity. I've been cancer free since my initial surgery, but nothing is promised.

Wishing all of you love, light, and peace as you navigate difficult waters.

Onward to the Appendix. It covers an encapsulation of Mark Lintern's Cancer Through Another Lens and the Resource Section.

Cancer Through Another Lens by Mark Lintern

Cancer Through Another Lens by Mark Lintern

Presentation references & synopsis:

Event Date: February 12th 2023

SYNOPSIS:

While scientists have made great progress against many diseases, cancer has not fared so well. Despite a monumental effort to understand the disease the mainstream *Somatic Mutation Theory* (SMT) hasn't delivered the results we were hoping for. As it stands the underlying cause of cancer remains unknown, which is why at least eight different theories of cancer co-exist. While researchers are working hard to find a solution, it should be noted that their efforts are being hindered by an incomplete understanding of the disease. Surely an effective treatment can only be realised once the underlying cause has been successfully identified. To that end we must continue to question what we think we know and remain open to new perspectives if we are to conquer this complex disease.

At present, the *Metabolic Theory* stands as the most accurate cancer theory currently available when evaluated against the Hanahan and Weinberg hallmarks of cancer. These are officially recognised as the main traits of the disease and are arguably the parameters most suited to assessing the validity of any theory – the more hallmarks that can be explained the more accurate a theory is deemed to be. To put this in context, the Metabolic Theory can explain nine of these 10 hallmarks and is close to explaining the remaining hallmark, whereas the mainstream Somatic Mutation Theory, also known as the *DNA Theory*, struggles to explain more than two. This indicates that DNA mutations are a symptom of the disease as opposed to the mechanism driving it, and that cancer is a metabolic disease driven by abnormal energy respiration. Given this, there is a strong case for offering metabolic treatments as standard care. The concern is that many in the field continue to claim that the DNA Theory is correct even though it remains an unproven theory, and that this will result in a continued reliance on DNA-based treatments that have been shown to be largely ineffective.

Recognising the shortcomings of placing all our faith in one unproven theory, leaders in the field continue to develop other theories to address the remaining aspects of the disease that the DNA Theory is struggling to account for. For instance, the Metabolic Theory has been complemented in recent years by the *Atavistic Theory* and the *Tissue Organisation Field Theory* (TOFT). The former seeks to explain why cancer cells revert to an old evolutionary form of metabolism (aerobic glycolysis) and how this results in an *epithelial-mesenchymal transition* (EMT) leading to an embryonic stem-cell-like phenotype. The latter asserts that carcinogenic insult results in the loss of suppressive growth signals in surrounding tissue leading to abnormal, invasive tumour growth.

Together these theories have greatly advanced our understanding and provide new treatment avenues that appear more successful than current standard of care treatments. However, there is a caveat. While the Metabolic Theory acknowledges the Warburg effect and it's clear that abnormal metabolism plays a pivotal role, there seems to be contention over the mechanism purported to be driving this condition. Professor Seyfried cites defective Oxidative Phosphorylation (OXPHOS) as the origin of cancer, however, OXPHOS has been shown to be operational to varying degrees in many cancers, while cells of the body such as endothelial cells, that rely heavily on glycolysis, do not become cancerous as a matter of normal function – indicating that some additional factor is required for cancer to form over and above a reliance upon glycolysis. Oncocytomas, which have defective OXPHOS, generate benign tumours as opposed to malignant cancers.

Regardless, Hallmark 7 (abnormal metabolism) is a crucial hallmark to account for because it appears to be the gateway to explaining the other nine hallmarks of cancer, all of which appear to result from the Warburg effect. This is why Professor Seyfried places so much emphasis on this aspect of the disease, he recognises that the Warburg effect is pivotal to explaining cancer. Determining the potential causes of the Warburg effect then, will likely lead to the identification of the underlying mechanism(s) responsible for driving the disease.

To this end, I have spent the last eight years investigating this link and collating the evidence for a plausible mechanism. The sum of this evidence suggests that carcinogenesis can be interpreted through a different lens entirely. I have documented my findings in a way that not only compliments the theories that already exist, but also provides an alternative explanation for the Warburg effect, as well as all nine other Hanahan and Weinberg hallmarks of cancer. In addition, this new interpretation of the science provides a unique explanation of at least 20 other cancer-related conditions, such as arginine auxotrophy, the reverse Warburg effect and chemotherapy resistance (see the RESULTS section below). This indicates that an entirely different mechanism is at play.

Intriguingly, this new perspective does not rewrite how we treat the disease from a metabolic point of view, far from it. In fact, it encompasses all the very same treatments advocated for by the Metabolic Theory, but it also highlights the need to consciously target an additional factor that many metabolic treatments are often inadvertently targeting. All that may be needed to treat cancer more effectively is to make minor adjustments to the metabolic approach.

To explain, I would like to shift your perspective of the disease momentarily. Nearly all mainstream theories view cancer through the same lens – the notion that it arises from a malfunction within the cell due to damage. Such a malfunction is thought to develop within the genome, within mitochondria, or within the surrounding tissue leading to a loss of suppressive growth signals. It is this breakdown in cell functionality that allegedly drives the disease. For instance, the DNA Theory claims that mutated DNA genes are responsible, the *Aneuploid Theory* asserts that abnormal chromosome formation is the driver, whereas the Metabolic Theory claims that faulty mitochondria trigger an energy switch that results in the conditions of cancer. All data is interpreted through this cell-malfunction lens where the cell itself is ultimately to blame. One could argue that currently only one overall theory of cancer exists – the *Cell Malfunction Theory* if you will, and that all mainstream theories are sub-theories within this paradigm. The contention between these theories lies in which part of the cell is faulty and therefore responsible. The problem for all these theories has been an inability to identify a pattern of damage that can account for the consistency of the disease.

What if the abnormal behaviour of a cancer cell is not a result of malfunction, but of suppression, where an external factor foreign to the cell influences cell death and growth mechanisms, leaving the cell no longer in full control?

In support of this concept, Ravid Straussman's pioneering work has illustrated that tumours used in laboratory experiments, which were previously thought to be sterile, harbour intracellular micro-organisms and a tumour-specific microbiome that interfere with cell functionality and drug effectiveness. Significantly, studies analysing the microbiome of oral cancer patients show that a particular type of micro-organism dominates, and that it can instigate most of the hallmarks we see in cancer. Recent evidence highlighting the direct influence of these micro-organisms in driving the disease has prompted Douglas Hanahan to update the hallmark list to include a 'Polymorphic microbiome' as part of the equation. And when searching for an answer to arguably the most pressing question in cancer research: '*What's the underlying cause of hallmark 7?*' studies confirm that, upon infection, pathogens instigate the Warburg effect – the Warburg effect is a natural anti-infection response.

Here, hiding in plain sight is a known cause for the Warburg effect, ignored up until now due to the common assertion that cancer results from faulty cell machinery. While the notion of cancer resulting from infection is not new, this cell suppression concept is unique and has yet to be explored by scientists. Currently, around 20% of cancers are associated with infection, but not in a suppressive capacity; rather, micro-organisms are thought to damage the cell leading to malfunction – and it is this malfunctioning cell machinery that is ultimately thought to be driving the disease, rather than the micro-organism per se.

Challenging this perspective, I'm proposing that it's the suppressive nature of the pathogen and its control over specific cell functions, such as cell death and cell growth mechanisms, that's driving the disease, not the random damage inflicted by infection or carcinogens. We now know that intracellular micro- organisms exist within tumours, that pathogens actively suppress tumour-specific cell functions in order to keep the cell alive so long as it's beneficial for their survival, and we know that the Warburg effect is triggered as part of an anti- microbial defence mechanism. During the infectious process the Warburg effect is actively sustained until the infection is eradicated regardless of oxygen availability. Failure to eradicate the infection provides an explanation for cancer's sustained reliance on glycolysis even in the presence of oxygen – the condition known as the Warburg effect. Ongoing damage to mitochondria results in an epithelial- mesenchymal transition that explains the reversion of regular cancer cells to one of a cancer stem-cell-like phenotype and accounts for unlimited growth. Latent survival within macrophages and lateral transfer of the pathogen between these immune cells also helps to explain metastasis, immune evasion, the ability of cancer to cross the blood brain barrier and why macrophages appear to play a dominant role in cancer progression.

When viewed through this suppressive lens all major aspects of the disease can be explained. For example, in terms of understanding carcinogenesis, scientists are struggling to explain how the random DNA damage caused by so many different toxic carcinogens could lead to the consistency of cancer. This is certainly an impossible task given that randomness cannot generate consistency. To explain how the consistency of cancer can develop from the apparent randomness of carcinogen damage, we have to consider that there must be other consistent conditions generated by all carcinogens – and that these conditions have been overlooked. When we investigate further, this is indeed what we find. All carcinogens generate at least four consistent conditions: a weakened immune response, chronic inflammation, overproduction of lactic acid and iron overload. This is a crucial point to acknowledge because these conditions shed light on the underlying cause:

A weakened immune system offers less resistance to infection.

Inflammation renders cells more vulnerable to pathogen invasion.

Lactic acid overproduction and iron overload feeds the infectious process and has the adverse effect of suppressing immune cells at the site of injury.

Essentially, carcinogens generate favourable conditions that facilitate infection – this toxic niche feeds these pathogens and provides a protective environment within which the efficacy of the immune response is greatly reduced. Add in the Warburg effect and suppression of cell death mechanisms, and we have the promotion of a proliferative state that can explain the initial stages of carcinogenesis.

As the infection is slow-growing and encased within the protective boundary of the tumour, the patient won't be aware of the infection until the tumour grows large enough to be noticed. Assuming that cell malfunction is driving these conditions has meant we've overlooked another possibility – that sustained infection by particular pathogens is stimulating this abnormal cell expansion. Naturally, the increased absorption of glucose feeds the pathogen while depleting glucose within the surrounding tissue. This further suppresses the immune response at the tumour site because immune cells require glucose to operate. This provides an alternative explanation for why glucose feeds the disease – in sustaining the voracious demand of the pathogen, the monopolising of available glucose simultaneously depletes and weakens the immune response, all while the proliferative state of aerobic glycolysis stimulates cell proliferation.

Acquisition of nutrients by the pathogen, such as pyrimidines, purines, methionine and arginine, forces the cell to absorb higher quantities of these nutrients to replenish those that are lost. In effect, the cell is operating on autopilot having lost control of cell growth and cell death mechanisms. As with glucose, glutamine receptors are also stimulated because glutamine is converted into many essential nutrients that need replenishing – incidentally, the pathogen in question utilises this glutamine by converting it to glucose in situations where glucose availability is scarce. The consumption of methionine by the pathogen explains why hypomethylation is a condition of pre-cancerous tissue and accounts for the random DNA damage that occurs in early-stage tumour development. Acquisition of arginine explains arginine auxotrophy and why arginine starvation therapy can be effective but can also render the tumour more aggressive.

Inhibiting these fuels has been shown to inhibit cancer cells. This alternative perspective proposes that this is not just because the cell requires them to survive, but because the pathogen also requires these same fuels to sustain the infection. This explains why the mechanism of apoptosis – which is currently thought to be broken – is once again initiated when anti-microbial drugs or anti-microbial plant compounds (bromelain, sulforaphane) are introduced to cancer cells. The pathogen is killed allowing mitochondria to regain control of cell death mechanisms, resulting in apoptosis. The apoptotic pathway was never faulty, just suppressed by the pathogen.

Viewing cancer through the lens of cell suppression enables us to re-interpret why certain treatments appear effective, and why the survival rate is so low with current standard of care. For instance: three of the four drugs used by the Care Oncology Clinic aimed at inhibiting metabolic pathways, are also strong anti- microbial drugs. Metformin, Atorvastatin and Mebendazole are all effective at killing the common pathogens involved, not to mention that the first two inhibit the fuels that these pathogens also require to sustain the infection. Hyperbaric oxygen therapy is also anti-microbial, as is 3BP (3-Bromopyruvate), Tamoxifen, Arimidex, Lovastatin and many more besides. Regarding chemotherapy, while the free radicals generated by initial chemotherapy treatment can eradicate a large portion of the infection and reduce initial tumour size, chemotherapy often fails because it generates the same inflammatory conditions that go on to feed the infection – namely, immune weakness, chronic inflammation, overproduction of lactic acid and iron overload. Not to mention that the cell's free-radical-producing capacity is diminished over time due to the damage inflicted, which incapacitates mitochondria. The stimulation of cancer stem cells also plays a key role too. This explains why chemotherapy treatment can initially have a dramatic effect at reducing a tumour, but wanes substantially over time, and can become detrimental in the latter stages of treatment.

For the first time it is possible to explain why natural-based compounds such as bromelain, sulforaphane, honey and even silver can selectively kill cancer cells – all are highly anti-microbial. This new perspective has enabled the explanation of many key aspects of the disease, which are listed below.

RESULTS – Aspects of cancer explained by cell suppression:

- All 10 Hanahan and Weinberg hallmarks
- Carcinogenesis

An alternative explanation is also provided for:

- Glucose, glutamine, lactate, fat, methionine, and arginine used as fuel by cancer cells.
- The Reverse Warburg effect
- Arginine auxotrophy
- Methionine auxotrophy – methionine dependence
- Hypomethylation
- Aneuploidy
- Chemotherapy resistance
- Iron's role in carcinogenesis
- The role of estrogen
- The role of nagalase
- The role of galectin-3
- Why antioxidant supplementation aids tumour development
- The role of CYP1B1 and the reason for its upregulation
- The role of macrophages in tumour progression

- The role of myeloid-derived suppressor cells in tumour progression
- The reason for T-cell suppression
- Why cancer is primarily a disease of old age
- Why cancer incidence is increasing
- Why childhood cancers exist
- Why cancer appears to run in the family

An alternative explanation can be made for the effectiveness of particular treatments:

- The Care Oncology Clinic treatment protocol
- Metformin
- 3BP
- Statins – Lovastatin, Atorvastatin, Fluvastatin
- Tamoxifen
- Gleevec
- Herceptin
- Artemisinin
- Melatonin supplementation
- Hyperbaric oxygen therapy
- Ketogenic diet
- Fasting

- Salvestrols and other plant antibiotic compounds
- Restriction of glucose, glutamine, fat, methionine, arginine, and estrogen

Abundant evidence supports a metabolic approach to treatment, detoxification of the cellular terrain, and re-balancing of the microbiome in conjunction with the addition of a targeted anti-microbial solution. Data indicates that such a solution would work synergistically to target the dominant infection, which is protected within the inflamed toxic environment of the tumour. This would allow mitochondria to re-instigate apoptosis, resulting in regression of the disease.

OBJECTIVES:

In partnership with the integrative cancer care charity Yes to Life, we are hosting an online debate with the aim of evaluating this new perspective. A select group of expert cancer scientists, clinicians and cancer survivors will be present and taking part directly in the discussion – as will an invited audience of hundreds of scientists, clinicians and other cancer specialists. The merit of this new perspective will be discussed and carefully evaluated in a non-combative, constructive scientific manner.

The objective is to generate awareness of this cell-suppression concept, while subjecting it to a high level of scrutiny to assess its validity. The event will stimulate debate within the cancer community, highlight the serious flaws within the accepted paradigm and its approach to treatment and draw attention to the Metabolic Theory and metabolic treatments. The intention is to stimulate a shift in perspective that is hoped will lead to improved survival outcomes for people with cancer, as well as more robust prevention strategies.

CONCLUSION:

Abundant evidence supports the proposition that cancer is a cell-suppression disease caused by an opportunistic pathogen that takes advantage of the conditions arising from chronic inflammation. Emerging data confirms the presence of a dysbiotic tumour-associated microbiome dominated by common pathogens.

When viewed through the traditional 'cell malfunction' lens, it becomes impossible to identify the cellular mechanism(s) responsible for the odd behaviour expressed by the cancer cell because the cell itself is not at fault. This explains why the Somatic Mutation Theory cannot identify cancer-specific mutations, and why the Cancer Genome Atlas data shows that mutations appear random – these mutations are symptoms resulting from the infectious process and the initial toxin exposure. Cell suppression also explains why mitochondria appear to re-instigate apoptosis when supplied with plant antibiotic compounds, honey or silver. This cell death mechanism is suppressed rather than faulty.

The abundant evidence supporting a cell-suppression mechanism for carcinogenesis, in combination with its ability to explain all major hallmarks of the disease, makes it clear that further investigation is warranted to determine the validity of this premise. Discussing its merits openly amongst experts in the field will allow it to receive the attention it deserves, and provides the opportunity for it to improve our understanding of cancer, and hopefully the survival outcomes for patients.

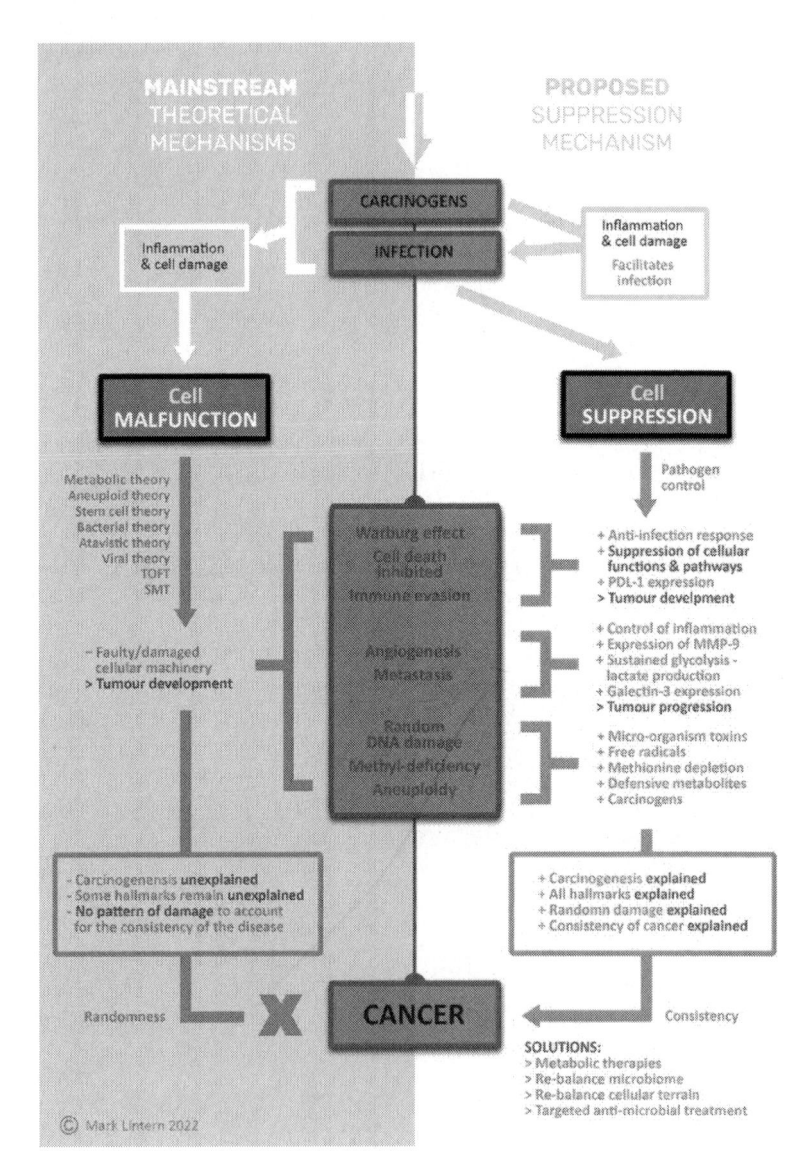

Cell malfunction vs cell suppression

ALIVE, SURVIVING MODERN ONCOLOGY   303

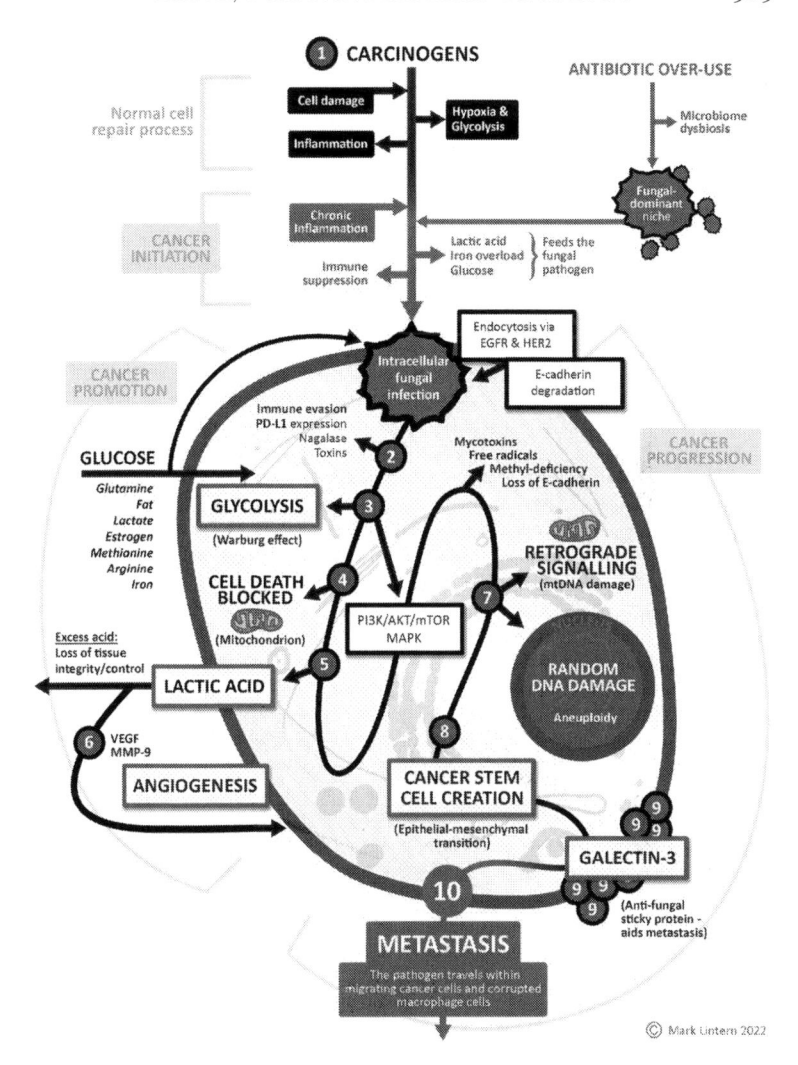

TUMOUR COMPOSITION
Cell suppression model

Lactic acid, iron overload, glucose depletion, chronic inflamation:
Creates a protective barrier around the tumour that suppresses immune cells, but feeds the pathogens present within the tumour mass, stimulating them to become aggressive and invasive.

Pathogen expansion:
Excess lactate fuels the infection which expands into surrounding tissue and dormant immune cells.

Reverse Warburg Effect:
Advancing infection stimulates the Warburg effect within the surrounding tissue. Peripheral tumour cells absorb the excess lactate as fuel.

Tumour-associated microbiome

Cell death inhibited, cell proliferation instigated, ineffective immune response

Cancer

Hypoxia + threat of infection:
Results in cells close to the infection, but not yet infected, instigating glycolysis, stimulating proliferation. It's only a matter of time before they become infected, and added to the tumour mass.

Blood vessel growth:
Blood vessels expand towards cells over-producing lactic acid. This corrosive environment, plus over-production of MMP-9, results in cells migrating into the bloodstream.

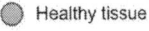

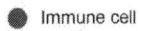

- ● Healthy tissue
- ● Immune cell
- ○ Warburg effect / anti-infection response > Tumour cell
- Intracellular pathogens > Cancer cells

ALIVE, SURVIVING MODERN ONCOLOGY

The fuels that feed cancer

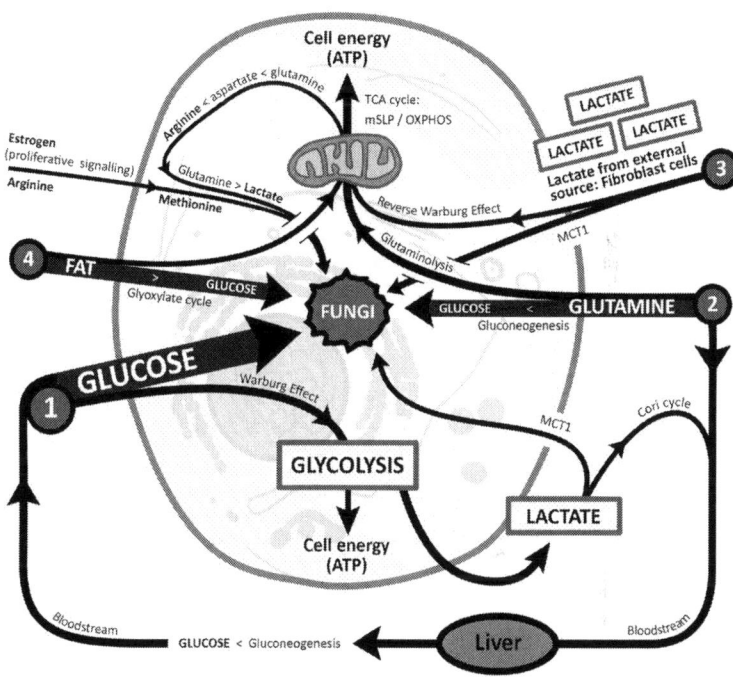

© Copyright MARK LINTERN 2023. All rights reserved.

REFERENCES for the above synopsis regarding infection and the Warburg effect:

1.   Timothy M. Tucey et al. *'Glucose Homeostasis Is Important for Immune Cell Viability during Candida Challenge and Host Survival of Systemic Fungal Infection.'* Cell Metabolism. 2018. doi.org/10.1016/j.cmet.2018.03.019

2.   Proal AD, VanElzakker MB. *'Pathogens Hijack Host Cell Metabolism: Intracellular infection as a Driver of the Warburg Effect in Cancer and Other Chronic Inflammatory Conditions.* Immunometabolism,2021;3(1):e210003. doi.org/10.20900/immunometab20210003

3.   Jorge Domínguez-Andrés, et al. *'Rewiring monocyte glucose metabolism via C-type lectin signalling protects against disseminated candidiasis.'* PLOS Pathogens. 2017. doi.org/10.1371/journal.ppat.1006632

4.   Cheng, Shih-Chin et al. *'mTOR- and HIF-1α-mediated aerobic glycolysis as metabolic basis for trained immunity.'* Science (New York, N.Y.). 2014. doi:10.1126/science.1250684

5.   Memorial Sloan-Kettering Cancer Centre. *'Sloan Kettering Institute Scientists Solve a 100-Year-Old Mystery about Cancer.'* January, 2021. https://www.mskcc.org/news/sloan-kettering-institute-scientists-solve-100-year- old-mystery-about? utm_source=Twitter&utm_medium=Organic&utm_-

campaign=012121MingLi-100- year-old- mystery&utm_content=Research&fbclid=IwAR0M7HU24J6RTLBXn-BHJ48B05cpYA CMLgIUJtHhFbuP7WsM5Z-0IXO-AE5A

6. Moyes, David L et al. '*Protection against epithelial damage during Candida albicans infection is mediated by PI3K/Akt and mammalian target of rapamycin signaling.*' The Journal of infectious diseases. June, 2014. doi:10.1093/infdis/jit824

7. Julian R Naglik, Sarah L Gaffen, Bernhard Hube. '*Candidalysin: discovery and function in Candida albicans infections.*' Current Opinion in Microbiology, Volume 52, 2019, Pages 100-109, ISSN 1369-5274, doi.org/10.1016/j.mib.2019.06.002.

8. Volling K, et al. '*Phagocytosis of melanized Aspergillus conidia by macrophages exerts cytoprotective effects by sustained PI3K/Akt signaling.*' Cellular Microbiology. 2011. doi: 10.1111/j.1462-5822.2011.01605.x

Resources

Resources:

I debated adding a resource section because many resources are fluid and a section such as this becomes dated quickly. Still, it holds critical information. Clearly, the books won't go anywhere. The online resources have been available throughout my journey and will continue to be updated with new information. For those reading the e-book, most links are embedded. For those reading the paperback, apologies. Most of the online integrative cancer groups maintain up-to-date resource lists.

Supplements:

Not all supplements are created equal. Taking high quality supplements is essential, which means not necessarily buying them off Amazon. You can get lucky and find high-quality brands on Amazon, Vitacost, Pure Formulas, or iHerb but why take a chance on products that may not be stored properly or may be counterfeits?

Basically, there are two ways to access practitioner-quality supplements: direct purchase or establishing care with a practitioner who has an account at one of many supplement wholesale shops.

The following is far from an exhaustive list. Many quality brands sell direct to the consumer, but it's best to get advice from an integrative healthcare practitioner before buying from any company.

U.S.

Fullscript (requires a practitioner) Fullscript also has a presence in Canada. (Maria Wessling Bachteal provides a discounted Fullscript dispensary to members of the Healing cancer Study Support group who have a US shipping address. Learn more here.

Emerson Ecologics (requires a practitioner)

Natura Health Products (requires a practitioner)

Happy Healing Store (source for fenbendazole, melatonin, and many other supplements)

PureBulk (high-dose melatonin and many bulk extracts)

Doctors Supplement Store (requires a practitioner) Maria Wessling Bachteal provides a discounted DSS dispensary to members of the Healing cancer Study Support group who have a US shipping address. Learn more here.

Jing Herbs (mushroom powders and Chinese herb blend powders. Use code mariab5 for 15% off.

Real Mushrooms (100% fruiting body extracts in capsules, powders, and specialty products. Maria provides a 20% discount through her affiliate link:

Kotuku Elixirs (reishi spore powder and other mushroom extracts and herbs) Use code FUNGI20 for 20% off.

U.K.

Your Health Basket (requires a practitioner)

Amrita (requires a practitioner)

Nutrilink (requires a practitioner)

Natural Dispensary

Turmeric and Honey

International

All Day Chemist (In India, a ~~good~~ source for Rx drugs if you can't get them from your MD. Prices are reasonable. Quality is sound.)

MCS Formulas (In the Netherlands). They ship to most countries free for purchases of 75 Euros or more and have cancer specific formulations that are more concentrated than you can get elsewhere. MCS Formulas donates a significant percentage of their funds to integrative cancer research.

To receive 5% off MCS prices, go to https://myhealingcommunity.com (Abbey Mitchell) or https://www.

healingnutritionofsonoma.com/recommendations (Maria Bachteal) to receive a discount code.

Biohawk (In Australia. He has products that have proven useful in cancer protocols.)

Clinics:

Many clinics are discussed in cancer groups across Facebook. Rather than list clinics, I'm going to note a few general principles.

1. Do not drain your life savings but don't forgo life-saving treatment just because it isn't covered by insurance. Results are far from guaranteed so get referrals from other patients before choosing a clinic. Spend what you can comfortably afford to lose. Discuss it with your family, decide on how much you'll spend, and stick with it. Consider a GoFundMe if money is tight, and you're convinced you need a particular treatment. None of us can do everything, but we give it our best shot. If you have scads of money, by all means research clinics. Some treatment might be covered by insurance, but don't bet on it. Alternative care can easily cost upward of $100,000/year.
2. This is tough to type—because I'm not quite there yet—but get comfortable with dying. You're not giving up, just developing a different perspective. Enjoy each day as it happens. It will relieve the enormous pressure we all feel to do EVERYTHING we can to eradicate every last cancer cell. I'm certainly

guilty of it. As my supplement list has grown and grown again, I've noticed nothing ever drops off it.
3. Understand the difference between "alternative and "integrative." Integrative practitioners like naturopathic oncologists, herbalists, licensed acupuncturists/TCM doctors, and integrative doctors can provide treatments to improve outcomes and reduce the side effects of chemo and radiation. It's important to research conventional options because newer targeted treatments and immunotherapies may offer good outcomes that could be improved by adding an integrative approach. The choice isn't always between "alternative" or "conventional." Integrative protocols combine the best of both.
4. If you're going to go the integrative/alternative cancer treatment route, do it early on before trying multiple rounds of chemo and radiation that weaken your body. I read a discussion between Dr. Mercola and Dr. Shields recently where they made that very point. Drs. Fung and Juneja do as well. Patients who come to them "fresh" had much better outcomes than patients who'd gone the standard of care route first.

Online Resources:

This is far from an exhaustive list. Every specific cancer has many online groups available, broader groups focus on alternative therapies for all cancer types. I belong to a couple related to uterine cancer. You don't have to dig very deep to find places full of relevant information.

Facebook is an excellent resource for online support groups. Research carefully and never take what other people write as fact. You will find much that is contradictory. Remember, cancer is an individual disease. Yours isn't like anyone else's, which makes genomic testing (both tumor and body genomics) so critical to finetune treatments.

MyHealingCommunity.com This is Abbey Mitchell's website and is affiliated with the Healing Cancer Study and Support Group on Facebook. Abbey works tirelessly to find answers for cancer patients. She is a rich source of knowledge.

Healingnutritionofsonoma.com This is Maria Wessling Bachteal's website She works with women who are in remission from breast cancer and other reproductive cancers. She also supports people with cancer through her Healing Nutrition of Sonoma Facebook page as well as being the co-developer (with Abbey Mitchell) of the Breast Cancer Pathways group on Facebook. Breast Cancer Pathways is an online resource for research on natural substances and off-label drugs.

Jane McLelland Off Label Drugs for Cancer on Facebook

Always Hope Cancer Protocol Support Group on Facebook

Fenbendazole Cancer Support Group on Facebook

Patient Led Oncology Trials on Facebook

Yes To Life (UK organization)

Radiant Healing Together (Circle and FB groups) This group, created by Amy Robinson, provides many resources including guided meditation and live meet-ups for breast cancer survivors

Radicalremission.com This is the website that grew from the books *Radical Remission* and *Radical Hope*.

PubMed is the government repository for all research articles published in journals worldwide. Input search terms and cull through what pops up. Be sure to set aside adequate time as PubMed searches can take hours.

Testing Companies:

Circulating Tumor Cells (CTCs)—used to predict risk of recurrence

Maintrac (Available in Europe and UK)

Cell *Search* (Available in US and Canada through various labs)

Signatera (Available in US and Canada, requires tumor cell and ongoing blood testing to check CTCs)

Personalized Cancer Treatments (typically require live tumor tissue)

Paris Test

Nagourney Cancer Institute

Weisenthal Cancer Group

Cancer Molecular Profiling (genomic mutations)

Tempus

CARIS

Guardant

Biotheranostics Cancer Type ID

Foundation One (most oncologists prefer this test because of wide acceptance by insurance companies but it's limited because it mainly identifies mutations covered by clinical trial drugs

Early Detection

Grail Galleri

Prenuvo Whole Body Scan

https://www.prenuvo.com/

Genetic Testing (inherited germ line mutations)

Consult genetic counselor through your physician

Epigenetic Testing (there are many. Here are a few used by integrative health practitioners because the results are considered well-validated by research.)

Nutrigenomic Testing

Nutrition Genome

DNA Life

Self Decode

Books:

In no particular order. There are so many others, but these are ones I've read and utilized along my journey. I found them empowering and inspiring.

The Metabolic Approach to Cancer: Integrating Deep Nutrition, the Ketogenic Diet, and Nontoxic Bio-Individualized Therapies by Nasha Winters ND

Mind Over Medicine by Lissa Rankin MD (She has a number of titles out, all are excellent)

How to Starve Cancer...And Then Kill It With Ferroptosis by Jane McLelland (Jane popularized the concept of blocking metabolic pathways.)

Breath: The New Science of a Lost Art by James Nestor (good for meditation practice)

Close to the Bone: Life-Threatening Illness as a Soul Journey, Jean Shinoda Bolen, M.D.

Questioning Chemotherapy by Ralph W. Moss Ph.D.

Life Over Cancer: The Block Center Program For Integrative Cancer Treatment by Keith Block MD

Naturopathic Oncology: An Encyclopedic Guide For Patients and Physicians, 4th Edition, by Neil McKinney (This is a classic, must have reference.)

EFT Tapping: Quick and Simple Exercises to De-Stress, Re-Energize and Overcome Emotional Problems Using Emotional Freedom Technique by Mike Moreland

Radical Remission: 10 Key Healing Factors from Exceptional Survivors of Cancer & Other Diseases by Kelly A. Turner (There is a companion volume, *Radical Hope*, that is also excellent.)

Ravenous, Otto Warburg, the Nazis, and the Search for the Cancer-Diet Connection by Sam Apple.

Love, Medicine and Miracles: Lessons Learned about Self-Healing from a Surgeon's Experience with Exceptional Patients by Bernie S. Siegel, MD (Dr. Siegel was one of the first to recognize that the "noisy" patients had far better survival rates and he encouraged active involvement in care.)

Cancer Care, The Role of Repurposed Drugs and Metabolic Interventions in Treating Cancer by Paul Marik MD. This book is a free download and available via this link. https://covid19criticalcare.com/reviews-and-monographs/cancer-care/

The Cancer Resolution? Cancer Reinterpreted Through Another Lens by Mark Lintern (only available in paperback from Amazon)

Notes

15. Eleanor Hall's Story

1. WebMD Editorial Contributors, Health Benefits of Black Garlic. Scroll down to "Fights Some Cancers." https://www.webmd.com/diet/health-benefits-black-garlic
2. A.S. Asom et al. Small cell cancer of the ovary, pulmonary type: A role for adjuvant radiotherapy after Carboplatin and etoposide? *Gynecological Reports*, Vol. 39, February, 2022, 011925. https://www.sciencedirect.com/science/article/pii/S2352578922000054#bb0015 Traditional Chinese Medicine is mentioned in the paragraph under the three pictures with black backgrounds.

About the Author

Ann Gimpel is a USA Today bestselling author. A lifelong aficionado of the unusual, she began writing speculative fiction a few years ago. Since then her short fiction has appeared in many webzines and anthologies. Her longer books run the gamut from urban fantasy to paranormal romance. Once upon a time, she nurtured psychology clients. Now she nurtures dark, gritty fantasy stories that push hard against reality. When she's not writing, she's in the backcountry getting down and dirty with her camera. She's published over 100 books to date, with several more planned for 2023 and beyond. A husband, grown children, grandchildren, and wolf hybrids round out her family.

Keep up with her at www.anngimpel.com or http://anngimpel.blogspot.com

If you enjoyed what you read, get in line for special offers and pre-release special reads. Newsletter Signup!

Also by Ann Gimpel

SERIES

Alphas in the Wild

Hello Darkness

Alpine Attraction

A Run for Her Money

Fire Moon

Bitter Harvest

Deceived

Twisted

Abandoned

Betrayed

Redeemed

Bound by Shadows

Scarred

Cursed

Promised

Cataclysm

Harsh Line

Warped Line

Cracked Line

Broken Line

Circle of Assassins

Shira

Quinn

Rhiana

Kylian

Grigori

Coven Enforcers

Blood and Magic

Blood and Sorcery

Blood and Illusion

Demon Assassins

Witch's Bounty

Witch's Bane

Witches Rule

Dragon Heir

Dragon's Call

Dragon's Blood

Dragon's Heir

Dragon Lore

Highland Secrets

To Love a Highland Dragon

Dragon Maid

Dragon's Dare

Dragon Fury

Earth Reclaimed

Earth's Requiem

Earth's Blood

Earth's Hope

Elemental Witch

Timespell

Time's Curse

Time's Hostage

Gatekeeper

Shadow Reaper

Rebel Reaper

Untamed Reaper

GenTech Rebellion

Winning Glory

Honor Bound

Claiming Charity

Loving Hope

Keeping Faith

Ice Dragon

Feral Ice

Cursed Ice

Primal Ice

Magick and Misfits (Fall and Winter 2020)

Court of Rogues

Midnight Court

Court of the Fallen

Court of Destiny

Rubicon International

Garen

Lars

Soul Dance

Tarnished Beginnings

Tarnished Legacy

Tarnished Prophecy

Tarnished Journey

Soul Storm

Dark Prophecy

Dark Pursuit

Dark Promise

Underground Heat

Roman's Gold

Wolf Born

Blood Bond

Wayward Mage

Hands of Fate

Jinxed

Hunted

Salvaged

Tiana

Wolf Clan Shifters

Alice's Alphas

Megan's Mates

Sophie's Shifters

Wylde Magick

Gemstone

Lion's Lair

Unbalanced

STANDALONE BOOKS

Branded, That Old Black Magic Romance (paranormal romance)

Edge of Night (short story collection, paranormal and horror)

Grit is a 4-Letter Word (nonfiction)

Heart's Flame (post-apocalyptic romance)

Icy Passage (science fiction romance)

Marked by Fortune (post-apocalyptic coming of age story)

Melis's Gambit (historical paranormal romance)

Midnight Magic (paranormal romance)

Red Dawn (post-apocalyptic paranormal romance)

Shadow Play (historical paranormal romance)

Shadows in Time (Highland time travel romance)

Since We Fell (contemporary romance)

Warin's War (paranormal romance)

Printed in Great Britain
by Amazon